genetic rounds

genetic rounds

A Doctor's
Encounters in
the Field That
Revolutionized
Medicine

Robert Marion, MD

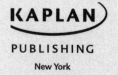

KAPLAN

PUBLISHING

New York

0321008640

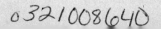

© 2010 Robert Marion, MD

Previously published in hardcover as Genetic Rounds (ISBN 978-1-60714-460-1)

Published by Kaplan Publishing, a division of Kaplan, Inc.
395 Hudson Street
New York, NY 10014

Printed in the United States of America

10 9 8 7 6 5 4 3 2

ISBN 978-1-60714-716-9

Library of Congress Cataloging-in-Publication Data

Marion, Robert.
Genetics rounds : a doctor's encounters in the field that has
revolutionized medicine / Robert Marion.
    p. ; cm.
ISBN 978-1-60714-460-1 (Hardcover)
1. Marion, Robert. 2. Medical genetics--United States--Biography. I.
Title.
 [DNLM: 1. Marion, Robert. 2. Genetics, Medical--Personal Narratives. 3.
Physicians--Personal Narratives. WZ 100 M3387g 2009]
 RB155.M345 2009
 616'.042092--dc22
 [B]
                              2009019110

Kaplan Publishing books are available at special quantity discounts to use for sales promotions, employee premiums, or educational purposes. For more information or to purchase books, please call the Simon & Schuster special sales department at 866-506-1949.

For Beth

CONTENTS

INTRODUCTION

NEARLY TEN YEARS AGO, when my daughter Dori was a senior in high school, she and I attended the Rye Youth Council's annual awards breakfast at a local church, where she was to receive one of the council's community service awards. As we took our seats at one of the tables, I looked around the room for familiar faces. My gaze settled on a family sitting at a neighboring table, an older couple and their son, a handsome boy who looked to be about the same age as Dori. Although I was certain I'd never seen this boy before, I was sure I knew his parents from somewhere; I just couldn't figure out where.

It took me a couple of minutes of staring and thinking to finally make the connection, and when I did, I was transported back more than 20 years, before their son was born, to what for both this couple and for me was another lifetime.

IN AUGUST 1980, I was a second-year resident in pediatrics at the Jonas Bronck Hospital in the Bronx. August was one of my elective months, so rather than working in the neonatal intensive care unit and further developing my already impressive peptic ulcer, or slaving away endless hours in the equally stressful pediatric emergency room, I was doing a rotation I really enjoyed, working in the Genetic Counseling Program at the Kennedy Center, a building adjacent to the Bronck.

I can't say for sure exactly when I realized that I wanted to be a geneticist. During college, I'd taken Introduction to Genetics and loved it. But I think that was due more to the fact that the course was taught by Dr. Timothy Lyerla, a terrific professor, than to the subject matter. (After interviewing hundreds of medical school applicants through the years about which college course they liked best and why, I've come to the conclusion that the teaching talent of the professor is the main reason students enjoy one particular course more than others.) As a senior, I did a semester of independent research with Dr. Lyerla, investigating some of the mysteries of Huntington disease, a neurodegenerative disorder that's inherited in an autosomal dominant manner (meaning that it's passed from affected parent to affected child). I enjoyed that research, but I can't say I liked it more than the independent work I did in ecology or invertebrate zoology, other areas of biology that had captured my interest during my undergraduate years.

I guess it was because of the comfort I'd attained with genetics as an undergraduate that, upon entering medical school, I sought out the staff of the Genetic Counseling Program. During my first year at the Albert Einstein College of Medicine, I did a mandatory community medicine project with the genetic counseling staff, and I was hooked. Before long, I was spending all my free time hanging around, trying to soak up as much about clinical genetics as I could. And so, by the time I was a resident, whenever people needed to locate me during one of my elective months, they didn't have to consult the schedule: they always knew exactly where to look.

In 1980, Thursdays were big days at the Genetic Counseling Program; on Thursday mornings, amniocenteses were performed. On most Thursdays, 20 or more procedures were done, each taking between 15 and 20 minutes. By 8:00 A.M. on those mornings, the waiting room would already be packed with pregnant women, most of them referred for testing because of advanced maternal age (which, for reasons that are still unknown, is associated with an increased risk of certain chromosomal abnormalities in the fetus), and their significant others, nervously anticipating their procedures. The tension in that room was always palpable. Some women focused on their fear of the needle; they couldn't begin to imagine how painful it was going to be to have a six-inch spinal needle plunged into the dark, secret recesses of their womb. But most women and their partners focused on the significance of the test's results: What would happen if, as a result of the probing of that needle into that secret place, they were to find that the fetus whose movements they were already feeling, whose images they had already seen on the monitor of an ultrasound machine, had Down syndrome, spina bifida, or some other serious condition? Faced with this information, what would they do? Would they choose to terminate the pregnancy at so late a date, after they had felt life, or would they continue the pregnancy, knowing that in five months they would become the parents of a child with a significant lifelong problem? It was a choice most couples never even wanted to consider, let alone one about which they'd have to make a timely decision.

Entering the waiting room that Thursday morning in early August, I was pleasantly surprised to see Dr. Sheldon Cohen sitting among the anxious assemblage. I'd known Dr. Cohen since my first semester of medical school. A member of the Einstein faculty, he'd taught part of the first-year course in pulmonary physiology. Later, when I'd been a third-year student, he'd been my preceptor during my internal medicine clerkship. A gifted teacher with a terrific sense of humor, Dr. Cohen had somehow been able to take some of the driest, most boring concepts in medicine and, like Dr. Lyerla during my undergraduate days, make them not only easy to understand but also enjoyable.

I walked over and said hello. Though clearly tense, he introduced me to his wife, Barbara, who was an anesthesiologist at one of the hospitals affiliated with Einstein, and tried to make some light conversation. Dr. Cohen (who had immediately ordered me to call him Sheldon) told me that Barbara, then in the 16th week of her first pregnancy, had been referred for the procedure by her obstetrician because at 36 she was considered to be of "advanced maternal age."

"You hear that?" he said to his wife with a smile. "We're here because you're old. I'm married to an elderly primip [woman in her first pregnancy]. Understand? You're old!"

"Oh yeah?" Barbara replied, smiling back. "Well, Sheldon, you're two years older than me, aren't you? If I'm old, what does that make you?"

Dr. Cohen was silent for a minute. "I hadn't thought of that," he finally said. "On second thought, maybe you're not so old."

About half an hour later, Barbara was called into the procedure room for her amnio. As usual during that month, it was my job to assist the obstetrician who performed the tap. While watching the sonogram, I gave the couple a running commentary as fetal parts whizzed by on the monitor's screen. "There's the head," I said.

"Looks like a cold front coming from the south," Sheldon replied.

"It does look like a weather map," I said. "By the way, that's the placenta," I continued, pointing to the screen, "attached to the lower portion of the uterus."

"Or it could be a line of thunderstorms moving through the region," Sheldon added.

"It's really amazing," Barbara said.

"There you can see the heart beating," I continued, pointing to the four-chambered view as it appeared on the screen. Both Sheldon and Barbara looked on in awe. No wisecrack followed this comment; I think that, even though the images, compared with today's sonographic pictures, were primitive, Sheldon realized for the first time that we were looking at his first child.

"These dark areas around the fetus represent pockets of amniotic fluid," I concluded. The sonographer chose one of those pockets, and using a black marker, I made a spot on Barbara's abdominal wall directly over that site.

While the obstetrician pulled on a pair of gloves, I opened the sterile tray that held the equipment needed for the tap. As we prepared, neither Barbara nor Sheldon made a sound; both seemed to be holding their breath. Even though they were both physicians, they were incredibly apprehensive.

The tap went off without a hitch. After gently cleaning the skin with an antibacterial solution, the obstetrician plunged the spinal needle directly through the black mark I'd made on Barbara's abdomen. Although she winced initially, the muscles of her abdomen quickly relaxed and clear amniotic fluid bubbled up through the needle's hub and began spilling onto Barbara's abdomen. Attaching a syringe to the hub of the needle, the obstetrician gently pulled back on the plunger until 30 cubic centimeters (one ounce) of fluid filled the chamber. The obstetrician pulled the needle out and covered the area with a gauze pad. Within seconds, Barbara was off the table and walking, with Sheldon's assistance, back to the waiting area. In another half hour, they were on their way out the door, understanding that it would take about two weeks until the results were ready.

As part of my elective, when things were quiet in the clinic, I spent time in the cytogenetics lab, where the amniotic fluid specimens were analyzed. One morning, Leslie Smith, the head cytogenetics technician, called me over to look at a chromosome spread. As I'd been trained, I looked through the microscope and counted the number of chromosomes present. I came up with 47. "That's one too many," I concluded, looking up from the microscope.

"And they said you'd never get this cytogenetics stuff," Leslie replied. "Can you tell which chromosome is trisomic?"

By then, I had become able to identify a few of the chromosomes according to their size and the unique pattern of light and dark bands that appeared after they were stained with Giemsa dye. Since trisomy 21, the chromosome abnormality that leads to Down syndrome, is by far the most common cause of an extra chromosome, I looked for the 21s first.

Identifying the characteristic pattern of dark and light bands, I counted three.

"Right. It's trisomy 21," Leslie told me. "I'll call downstairs. They'll have to get this couple in as soon as possible for counseling."

She picked up the phone and dialed the number of the clinic. I heard her say to the genetic counselor who answered: "Barbara Cohen is carrying a fetus with Down syndrome. The report will be finished later this afternoon."

I was in the room later that day when the medical geneticist who was head of the program told Sheldon and Barbara that their fetus had Down syndrome. I watched the tears come to their eyes. I heard their questions—about medical problems the baby might have, about longevity, about developmental issues that occur in children with Down syndrome, about the certainty of the diagnosis—and listened as the geneticist and the genetic counselor, trying to provide answers as nonjudgmentally as possible, patiently answered each one of them: Babies with Down syndrome are more likely to have a group of medical problems—about 40 percent have congenital heart disease, approximately 10 percent have intestinal problems and orthopedic problems, and many develop hypothyroidism and other endocrine problems. With good care, individuals with Down syndrome can live into their sixties and seventies. All individuals with Down syndrome have some degree of intellectual disabilities, which range from mild to severe. (And because an extra copy of chromosome 21 was present in every cell analyzed, the diagnosis of Down syndrome in the fetus was certain.)

Although this was the first time that I'd ever been involved with a patient who was an acquaintance of mine, at no time did I make eye contact with either Sheldon or Barbara; at no time did either of them make eye contact with me. After more than an hour, they left the office still crying, with Barbara clutching the card of an obstetrician who specialized in second-trimester terminations of pregnancy.

SEVEN MONTHS PASSED. In March 1981, I was scheduled for the second month of elective time during my junior residency year and, neither surprisingly nor unexpectedly, decided to spend yet another month at the Genetic Counseling Program. At a little after eight on the morning of the third Thursday of that month, Sheldon and Barbara Cohen entered the waiting room.

I hadn't seen either of them since they'd left the session back in August, but I could pretty much imagine what the last six months had been like for them. They'd obviously chosen to terminate the pregnancy, most likely via a dilatation and evacuation, a procedure in which Barbara's cervix was artificially dilated and the contents of her uterus were removed using a vacuum-like instrument. After recovering, Barbara had become pregnant again and was now here for another amniocentesis. Whether the emotional scars from the termination had healed, I could not tell. But on that morning in March, when I went to say hello to them, the Cohens were barely able to speak. Sheldon told me that they had mentioned this new pregnancy to no one and would continue to be tight-lipped about it until after the results of the amnio were back.

I understood that even choosing to try again to have a baby

must have been a difficult decision for the Cohens: because they had already had a fetus with Down syndrome, their risk of having another pregnancy complicated by a chromosome abnormality was increased over the general population.

Once again the amnio procedure went well. As I had done the first time, I began to describe the features of the fetus as they appeared on the screen, which had become kind of my trademark (I'm not sure whether anyone else ever took couples on a guided tour of their fetus during a sonogram), but neither Sheldon nor Barbara would look at the images; neither could risk bonding with this fetus or even acknowledge its existence until they knew its chromosomes were normal.

March ended, and I was working in the outpatient department in early April when the analysis of the chromosomes was completed. I was calling Leslie in the lab every day to find out the Cohens' results; finally, after 12 days, the results were in.

"It's normal," she told me, and I felt a weight lift off my shoulders. "A normal boy," Leslie concluded.

I HADN'T SEEN Sheldon or Barbara Cohen again until that morning when Dori and I were sitting at the table at the Rye Youth Council's award breakfast. After doing the math, figuring out how long it had been since that second amniocentesis, I realized that the handsome young man sitting between the Cohens, who, now that I looked more closely, had Sheldon's nose and Barbara's eyes, was undoubtedly the product of Barbara's second pregnancy.

By the time all of this had gone through my mind, the award ceremony had begun. More than 30 high school juniors and seniors were honored that morning, and Dori's award was the next-to-last one presented. I looked on with pride as her name was called and she rose to accept her plaque. But I also felt an unusual sense of pride when Jonathan Cohen's name was called as the winner of the last honor, the Rye Youth Council's Outstanding Citizen Award, and the young man sitting between Sheldon and Barbara rose and walked to the front.

After the ceremony ended, I walked up to the Cohens to say hello. Struck by the same problem I'd had when I first saw them, neither Sheldon nor Barbara could immediately place me. But when I said that, having last seen him on the screen of an ultrasound machine, it was nice to see how Jonathan had turned out, they immediately remembered who I was.

We spent a few minutes making small talk. Sheldon told me he'd left the Albert Einstein College of Medicine years before to join a private practice in the area. Barbara had retired from her work as an anesthesiologist just before Jonathan's birth and had spent the past 17 years caring for the couple's now three children. Eventually, both the Cohens and I got pulled in other directions and, after wishing one another the best, we separated. Not once during the minutes we spent together did any of us mention that afternoon in August 1980 when they heard the news from the medical geneticist about the extra chromosome; not once did the terms *Down syndrome* or *amniocentesis* come up. As I said before, it was as if the events surrounding Barbara's first pregnancy belonged to another life.

This episode is not unusual. Because of the nature of my work, because of the information I require and the data my investigations generate, I frequently delve into areas of my

patients' lives where friends, relatives, and other professionals cannot or choose not to go. Clinical genetics may be one
of the most private of all specialties in medicine. Although I
don't always feel comfortable with it, we clinical geneticists
spend a great deal of time rooting around in the closets of
the people who come to see us, visiting and examining the
skeletons that hang there, using the information that those
skeletons provide to help our clients make decisions about
their own family planning. As a result, I get to know about
the uncle with mental retardation whose existence, by virtue
of his having been institutionalized since early childhood, has
been kept a secret by the family; I get to review the autopsy
report of the baby with cyclopia and other congenital anomalies who, because the truth was believed to be too grotesque,
was said by his mother to have been stillborn due to a knot
in the umbilical cord; and, in the case of the Cohen family, I
got to be involved when Barbara's first pregnancy ended tear-
fully in a termination, something that she and her husband
probably had never disclosed to anyone, including Jonathan or
their other children. Because of this, medical genetics is like
no other medical specialty.

IT'S NOW BEEN nearly 30 years since I graduated from medical school. Back in 1975, the year Dr. Sheldon Cohen was trying his best to make pulmonary physiology interesting to
my classmates and me, genetics was little more to us than a
means to an end, a course my classmates and I had to pass in
order to do what we'd all really come to medical school to do,
that is, to take care of patients. Few of us took genetics very

seriously; most of my classmates memorized the facts, passed the exam, and promptly forgot virtually everything about the subject. And back in the 1970s, there was no problem with that approach: genetics was nothing more than a minor, insignificant subspecialty of pediatrics. (I like to tell students that this was exactly why I chose to become a geneticist: I was looking for something small and insignificant!)

But this all changed dramatically in the 1980s, when a major revolution occurred in genetics. With the development of a whole armamentarium of techniques, researchers became able to dissect the human genome. First, the locations of genes could be mapped to specific chromosomes. Next, the sequence of bases, the building blocks of the DNA molecule, could be analyzed for specific genes, and errors within the sequence, the so-called mutations that have been suspected of causing the disease processes, could be identified. Eventually, the defects in the proteins produced by those mutated genes could be found and some ideas about why such a change could produce a specific disease entity could be postulated.

This work culminated in 2001, with the announcement that, through the combined efforts of the Human Genome Project, a federal initiative supported by the U.S. Department of Energy and the National Institutes of Health, and Craig Ventor's privately owned Institute for Genomic Research, the complete human genome had been sequenced. And since that time, our knowledge of the genome has grown almost exponentially. In the past few years, I've repeatedly told my colleagues (half jokingly) that everything in medicine is genetic! But the truth is actually close to this statement: virtually all chronic disorders that occur in humans—including cancer, Alzheimer disease, schizophrenia, coronary artery disease, hypertension, diabetes, alcoholism, and asthma—are conditions in which a genetic predisposition combines with environmental factors to trigger a pathologic response. As a result, my classmates who failed to learn the basics of genetics and since graduation have treated the field as nothing more than a minor subspecialty have found themselves at a significant loss. And in the next quarter century, this knowledge will be harnessed to forever change the way medicine is practiced: new technology will allow us to diagnose and treat human diseases before they have even declared themselves, forever changing medicine from a field that is reactive (waiting for symptoms to develop and then treating those symptoms) to one that is proactive (taking steps to change the environment so that the conditions never occur). Truly, genetics has become so important that it is not inaccurate to say that, in contrast to the way things were when I was in medical school in the late 1970s, pediatrics—in fact all of medicine—is now nothing more than a small, insignificant subspecialty of genetics!

But as in many dramatic and sweeping changes in medicine, the technology that has led the way in the genetic revolution has far outstripped our ability to deal ethically with the advances. Sure, we can test a 35-year-old man whose father and grandmother died of complications of Alzheimer disease to see if he's inherited the *APOE E4* haplotype, a genetic variation commonly associated with the disorder, but what help does this provide? Without a treatment, without even strong evidence that inheriting this haplotype will with certainty lead to the development of dementia later in life, we are doing nothing more than sentencing him to years of anxiety and concern. And how about the 20-year-old woman whose mother and grandmother died of breast cancer in their early forties and who wants to know if she, too, is at risk for the same fate? Once we've done the blood work and found that she's carrying a mutation in the *BRCA1* gene, a finding that identifies her as having an up to 85 percent chance of developing breast cancer and a 30 percent chance of developing ovarian cancer at some point during her life, how should she be managed? To minimize her risk, should she immediately undergo bilateral mastectomies and a hysterectomy with removal of her ovaries? Should she be monitored closely and have these procedures after she's had children? Or should we just monitor her? And what of the psychological effect of having to live her life with this knowledge? Are we justified in imposing this on her without really any good sense of the best course of action to pursue? How do we support her psychologically? And if we decide that testing without having the ability to know for sure how best to treat her if she's positive for the mutation is not justified, is it ethical not to offer a test she is asking to have performed? Such questions, though difficult to answer, are posed every day in the life of the clinical geneticist.

The essays in this book are intended to provide some insight into the roles clinical geneticists play, describing the human side of the genetic revolution. The essays can be grouped into three types: (1) those that deal with some of the ethical dilemmas I've faced over the years, (2) those that explore some of the mysteries I've been asked to solve in some of the patients

I've seen, and (3) those that look at some aspects of life in academic medicine. (Due to the nature of our work, we clinical geneticists can exist only in large academic centers; hence, whether we like it or not, if we want to work as clinical geneticists, we have to spend our time in the ivory tower, which can lead to some pretty bizarre situations!) Through these essays, I hope you will come away with a feel for what my professional life is like today.

A note of caution: the essays that follow have been written over the past 20 years. Since their creation, since the time I saw the patients whose stories are detailed here, an enormous amount has changed in the technology available for diagnosing and treating these conditions. As an example, in "Relics," in order to test Mrs. Kennedy's fetus, it was necessary to have a sample of DNA from Sarah, the Kennedys' deceased first child. Today, direct DNA analysis for spinal muscular atrophy, in which we can look directly for mutations in the gene that cause the disease, is readily available, preventing us from needing tissue from the affected child (and therefore alleviating the horror experienced by her parents as we tried to find a way to help). But this is not designed to be an up-to-date textbook on clinical genetics; providing current information about diagnosis and treatment is not the point here; rather, it is the human side of the doctor–patient interactions that is important.

When I graduated from medical school, I had a good idea of what career path I wanted to follow. I didn't know exactly what I'd be doing 30 years later, but I knew I wanted to be a clinical geneticist. Although I've managed to attain that goal, the experience of working in this field for all these years has affected me, changed me, made me less idealistic and more jaded. For sure, the "me" of 30 years ago would be surprised by the values, emotions, and concerns of the "me" of today. Through the essays that follow, different aspects of how I approach patients and families will become apparent. Some of the changes have been good; many have not. I'll have much more to say about the effect that 30 years in practice have had on me in the Afterword.

AUTHOR'S NOTE

ALTHOUGH THE ESSAYS in this book are all based on my interactions with patients and families over the past 20 years, the names of people and the institutions in which they were seen have been changed in order to protect anonymity. Most of the action takes place at institutions called the Children's Hospital, Mt. Scopus Medical Center, Jonas Bronck Hospital, University Hospital, and Garwood Children's Hospital; these are not the real names of these institutions. In addition, for further protection, both identifying characteristics and specifics of our interactions may have also been altered. The events may not have occurred in the exact order or at exactly the same time as depicted, but all the medical details are accurate.

A number of these essays have previously been published, in somewhat different form, in the following publications: *Hippocrates* (Introduction); *Discover* ("A Case of Abuse," "The Baby Who Stopped Eating," "No Sweat!" "The Right Place, the Right Time," and "'Something's Bothering Me About This Baby'"); *The American Journal of Medical Genetics* ("Failing A.C.," "Scotty's Funeral," "The Christmas Present," "Erin, Before I Knew Her," and "The Skeleton in Mr. Anderson's Closet");

I. Edward Alcamo, ed., *Encounters in Microbiology,* Boston: Jones & Bartlett, 2001 ("The Baby Who Stopped Eating"); and *E=MD²: The Alumni Magazine of the Albert Einstein College of Medicine* ("Two Miracles, One Year Later" and the Afterword).

Finally, I'd like to thank Don Fehr and the amazing Rachel Bergmann at Kaplan for their editorial assistance; Dominique Polfliet, production editor par excellence, for her role as this book's midwife; and Janet Renard for her incredible copyediting. To Diana Finch, my literary agent, who has been there for me through thick and thin for the past 25 years, a big thank-you. Thanks also to my wife, Beth, and my children, Dori, Davida, and Jonah, for their understanding during the many hours over the years I worked on these essays. And of course, many thanks to my patients and their families, both those whose lives are chronicled in the pages of this book and those whose stories don't appear here, for allowing me to be a part of their lives.

CHAPTER 1

Failing A.C.

O NE ROLE OF medical geneticists is to serve as patient advocates. In their struggle to survive in a society that discriminates against people because of the way they look or act, the infants, children, and adults for whom I provide care clearly need my help. But sometimes, because of the complex interactions I have with different patients, I wind up being placed in the confusing position in which acting as an advocate for one patient might jeopardize my standing with another. Such a situation occurred when Ms. Sheridan brought her son, A.C., to see me for his monthly follow-up visit.

THE WAITING ROOM was nearly empty when Ms. Sheridan pushed A.C.'s stroller through our center's front door. Only one person was seated there when the Sheridans arrived, a young, pregnant African American woman who was waiting to see Carol Stern, one of our genetic counselors. Upon seeing Ms. Sheridan and her son, I gave them a rousing greeting.

"Say hello to Dr. Marion," Ms. Sheridan ordered A.C.

Without changing the expression on his face, without shifting or focusing his scarred, bulging eyeballs (which protruded so much that his eyelids had to be partially sutured shut by an ophthalmologist), A.C. waved to me as best he could, flapping his left hand and fingers slightly, the movements of the limb severely restricted by the bony fusion that permanently froze his radius, ulna, and humerus into a flexion contracture of the elbow.

I waved back at the boy and told his mother I'd be with them in a few minutes. Then I returned to my office to finish filling out the lab slips for the blood work I'd drawn from my previous patient.

After taking a seat opposite the desk of Billie Stein, our secretary, Ms. Sheridan unbuttoned A.C.'s coat and pulled off his fancy, colorful stocking cap to expose the boy's towering, lopsided skull. Working like a well-trained respiratory therapist, she quickly produced a catheter from the portable suction machine that lay hidden under the seat of the boy's specially designed infant stroller. As she plunged the catheter into the boy's tracheostomy (a surgically created opening in the neck to allow breathing), I heard the young prenatal patient, who was sitting off to the side and carefully observing the boy's striking deformities, ask A.C.'s mother, in a somewhat panicked voice, "What happened to your baby?"

Ms. Sheridan didn't answer. Knowing what was likely to happen next, I left my paperwork and nearly jumping out of my desk chair, ran into the waiting area, grabbed A.C.'s stroller, and began wheeling it into my office. "Come on in," I said to

Ms. Sheridan, who, I could see, was fuming. I was just barely able to get the door closed behind me before she exploded.

"Why can't people mind their own business?" she said, shaking her head.

"I see it's still happening," I said.

"All the time, Dr. Marion, all the time," Ms. Sheridan replied as she lifted A.C. from the stroller and put him on her lap. The boy stared up at his mother's face through those proptotic eyes. "Wherever I go, whenever I take A.C. out with me, in the street, in stores, everywhere. I don't mind so much when little kids do it. I understand they just don't know any better. But when it's an adult, like that woman out there, there's just no excuse for that."

"What do you tell people when they say things to you?"

"I tell them to mind their own business," she replied, "That's usually enough to get them to turn their heads away. I know A.C. looks different from everybody else. But still, there's no need to be rude."

"I agree completely. But you have to understand, when people see a kid like A.C. for the first time, they just don't know how to act. Even your family had trouble. But after I explained that A.C.'s problems were caused by a change in a gene, they seemed to understand."

"I know A.C. sets off a whole bunch of bells in people's heads," she responded. "But knowing it doesn't make it any easier."

"And it probably never will," I said, taking the boy from his mother and placing him on my own lap. "But unfortunately that's life: there's nothing we can do to fix it; all we can do is get used to it. Now, how has A.C. been since last month?"

HAVING BEEN BORN with a condition called Pfeiffer syndrome type III, a rare but devastating collection of unusual congenital malformations, A.C. required care from a team of medical and surgical specialists, including representatives from neurosurgery; plastic surgery; orthopedics; otorhinolaryngology (ear, nose, throat—ENT); ophthalmology; gastroenterology; endocrinology; and developmental pediatrics. Attempting to serve as the quarterback of this team of specialists, trying to simplify A.C.'s care and ensure that no problem fell through the system's cracks, I met with A.C. and his mother at least once a month to review the previous month's events, to answer Ms. Sheridan's questions, and to try as best as I could to coordinate the boy's care.

We started reviewing A.C.'s recent medical history, attacking one problem after another. I had finished getting updates on his routine health care maintenance (aside from his underlying condition, A.C. was in excellent health) and neurosurgical status (thus far, A.C. had undergone two craniofacial reconstructive surgical procedures, major operations designed to open the prematurely closed sutures of his skull, structures that normally remain patent until one year of age but that, because of his underlying condition, were fused by the time A.C. was one month old, severely limiting the space A.C.'s brain had available for growth; within weeks of both operations, A.C.'s sutures had re-fused, and now, six months after his last procedure, further surgery was being considered), and I was reviewing ENT (because of bony anomalies of his nose and throat that prevented him from being able to breathe, A.C. had required the placement of a tracheostomy in the newborn period) when my office intercom rang.

"Bob, you'd better come out here," I heard Billie say when I picked up the phone. "We have an emergency."

Telling Ms. Sheridan I'd be back in a few minutes, I handed A.C. to her, rose, and exited from the room.

I HEARD THE crying as soon as I entered the waiting area. It was loud and emotional and coming from Carol's office.

"What's wrong?" I asked Billie.

"That woman who was sitting out here when A.C. came in," the secretary said. "As you can hear, she's upset."

I knocked on the genetic counselor's door and quickly entered. Sitting at her desk, Carol was gently hugging the crying young woman, trying her best to comfort her.

"What's wrong?" I asked again.

"This is Ms. James. Ms. James, this is Dr. Marion," Carol began, still hugging the young woman. Then to me, she continued: "Ms. James is upset because of something that happened while she was out in the waiting room."

I nodded and asked why she'd come to see us in the first place.

"Ms. James is 21 years old and this is her first pregnancy," Carol told me. "In the prenatal clinic, she was found to have an elevated serum AFP."

AFP, short for *alpha-fetoprotein,* is, as the name implies, a protein produced during fetal life; it is detectable in the mother's blood and can be used as a screening test for various birth defects; when the maternal serum AFP is low, it can be a sign that the fetus has a chromosomal abnormality such as Down syndrome. AFP is therefore used as part of the so-called quad screen; when it's elevated, as it was in the case of Ms. James, it may be a sign that the fetus has one of a series of defects in the fetal skin, the most common of which is spina bifida.

"We did a sonogram today which showed that the fetus had no detectable anomalies. It turned out that Ms. James's dates were a little off; she's three weeks further along than she thought. I recalculated the AFP value based on the new dates, and it turns out that she's now within the normal range, so there's really nothing for her to worry about. Unfortunately, while I was on the phone getting the sonogram report, she was sitting in the waiting room and I guess she met A.C.—"

"That baby . . . that baby . . . ," was all Ms. James could manage through her tears.

Without considering what I was saying, I launched into a response designed to put Ms. James at ease. "That baby has a very rare condition. In all of recorded medical history, fewer than 50 babies have been reported to have had the condition."

"But what if my baby has the same thing?" Ms. James asked.

"Like I said, Ms. James, what A.C. has is very rare," I replied. "Because it's so rare, it's very, very unlikely that your baby could have the same thing."

"Ms. James, you just had a detailed sonogram that showed that your baby looks fine," Carol said reassuringly, and I nodded my head in agreement. "If your baby had this same condition, there would have already been signs that things weren't going well: the eyes would have looked bulgy, the head shape would have been abnormal, things like that. The fact that none of these features were found tells us that we can be pretty sure that your baby doesn't have this condition."

"But that sonogram could be wrong, couldn't it?"

"The doctor who looks at the sonogram is very good," I replied calmly. "She has a lot of experience looking at fetuses, and I trust her a lot. If she didn't find any of the problems Carol just mentioned, it would be very, very unlikely that your baby has this same condition."

With the woman now calmer, Carol told me that I could leave, that she'd continue speaking with Ms. James. Taking a deep breath, I returned to my office and, after apologizing to Ms. Sheridan (who, I'm almost certain, understood perfectly well where I'd been and what I'd been doing), picked up where we'd left off.

By the time I'd finished examining A.C. and Ms. Sheridan was pushing her son's stroller out through the waiting room's door, Ms. James had already departed. Afterward, Carol told me that she'd managed to get the woman to smile before she left. Since that visit to our office, Carol and I have spoken with Ms. James a few times; to date, her pregnancy has continued on without further complication.

It was only later, after I'd finished with my patients for the day and was sitting at my desk, completing my paperwork, that I began to feel angry with myself. In my trying to comfort Ms. James, I had failed A.C. As the boy's doctor, it had been my duty to try to educate that woman. I should have told her that although A.C. might look different on the outside, below the surface he was a child just like any other child, a human being who was loved by his mother, by his family, and by his doctors in the same way she would love the baby that was currently growing and developing inside her womb. As A.C.'s advocate, as an advocate for all patients who looked or acted differently from what was accepted as normal, I should have told her that it was wrong to judge a person simply on the basis of how he or she looked, wrong and discriminatory, as discriminatory as it might have been for white America to judge Ms. James's parents and grandparents simply on the basis of their skin color.

I could have told her these things, I should have told her these things, but the fact was that I hadn't. I was more concerned with reassuring her, with calming her hysteria, than I was with attempting to educate her, and in so doing I had let down A.C. and his mother. My failure may have been subtle, and it may have been completely unknown to the Sheridans, but I understood it; I knew I had done it, and it bothered me. And as I write this, the incident bothers me still.

Postscript

AS I WRITE THIS, A.C. Sheridan is now 16 years old. As far as I know, he is the oldest person in the universe with Pfeiffer syndrome type III. His case has appeared in the medical literature at least three times.[1]

As the years have passed, we've learned a lot about the genetic basis of the condition that affects A.C. We've learned that, like most people who have one of the three types of Pfeiffer syndrome (which range from mild to severe), A.C. has a mutation in a gene called *FGFR2*. His particular mutation is *Trp290Cys;* to describe this in more straightforward language, I'll need to explain a little bit about molecular genetics.

Genes, the blueprints that tell the body how to form, do their work by "ordering" cells to use their machinery to make proteins; the proteins, composed of amino acids, are created using the instructions that are inherent in the sequence of bases, the building blocks that form the DNA. The proteins are the workhorses that carry out the work of the gene. A change in the base sequence may lead to a change in the amino acid sequence, altering the resulting protein, preventing it from working properly, leading to a series of symptoms and signs. In A.C.'s case, a single base change in the DNA that composes the coding sequence of the *FGFR2* gene has caused a substitution of the amino acid cysteine for the amino acid tryptophan at the position that corresponds to the 290th amino acid in the protein produced from instructions from *FGFR2*. This single base change, out of the total of 3 billion bases that make up the human genome, has caused the protein to be so abnormal that it has resulted in the severe malformations with which A.C. was born.

We've learned that the mutation in A.C. occurred spontaneously in the sperm or the egg that formed him, as testing of his parents, who have no features of Pfeiffer syndrome, revealed that neither of them had the same mutation present in A.C. We learned that the protein produced by the *FGFR2* gene is fibroblast growth factor receptor type 2, one of a family of at least 22 related proteins that regulate cell proliferation, differentiation, and migration through a variety of complex pathways that are important in formation of blood vessels, wound healing, limb development, and other important processes. We've learned that these receptors act in concert with another type of protein, fibroblast growth factors, during very early development.

But, as is the case with most genetic conditions, although we've learned all of these facts about the molecular basis of this disease, we are still virtually powerless to do anything to help A.C. or to prevent this condition from occurring in the first place. So A.C. carries on as he always has, while we, his doctors, feel simultaneously smug about how much we know and frustrated because of our inability to use any of this great knowledge to do anything to improve his life. Unfortunately, this is a common theme in the practice of clinical genetics.

Although his doctors know all this stuff about Pfeiffer syndrome, A.C. himself doesn't. Developmentally impaired, he began to walk on his own at the age of 10, began speaking in recognizable words about a year later, and is still not toilet trained. Despite numerous neurosurgical procedures and plastic surgeries, his presence in our waiting room, on the bus, or in any place outside his family's apartment continues to evoke the same reaction that occurred when Ms. James saw him as an infant. As a result of these reactions, and the continuing sensitivity of his mother to his plight, A.C. has never attended school (he receives home instruction), never had a friend or companion who was not a member of his family, and never taken a vacation or gone anywhere outside his neighborhood. A.C.'s mother is private about her son's condition, a stance many families take after the birth of a child with malformations.

Through the years, I've encouraged Ms. Sheridan to allow A.C. to spend time with children his own age (after all, he doesn't seem to be adversely affected by the stares and whispering; he is as well-adjusted as he could possibly be, considering the isolated and restricted environment in which he's been raised), but she has refused to let her son out of her sight.

"Dr. Marion," she tells me, "A.C. is a miracle. He's my miracle, and he wouldn't be here today if it wasn't for my watching out for him the way I do. If he's in school, is his teacher going to let me sit there with him and take care of him? I don't think so! And if I'm not there to watch out for him and take care of him, who's going to protect him? No one!"

I try to convince her that we have to consider what's in the best interest of A.C., but at some level I know she's right. He's alive today only because of the excellent care she has provided for him. And chances are that he'll live a long time, at least as long as his mother is around to hover over him and provide for his every need. But what will happen when, due to infirmity or death, she is no longer around to care for her son? I have no answer to this question. And, unfortunately, this is a huge unanswered question that occurs in the lives of many of my patients.

CHAPTER 2

A Case of Abuse

You COULD TELL a lot about the Moore family by the way its members assembled themselves around my office that afternoon. Melissa, who had just celebrated her first birthday, was sitting on the floor, playing with an assortment of blocks and other toys her parents had brought for her. Her mother, Lisa, was sitting on a couch, three feet away from her daughter. At the other end of the room, sitting on a chair close to my desk, was Barry, Melissa's father. At no time during the more than one hour we spent together did Lisa and Barry make eye contact or speak directly to each other. At no time did Melissa attempt to crawl toward either of her parents, nor did she express the need to be comforted by her mother or to sit on the lap of her father. This wasn't exactly the kind of behavior one would expect from a family during their first visit to the medical geneticist's office.

I knew full well why the Moores were acting this way. Although this was the first time we'd met in person, I'd become involved in Melissa's case six months before. Back then, I'd received a call from their pediatrician, Dr. Jeremy Stanger. Jeremy and I were residents together, and whenever he has a concern about the possibility of a genetic disorder in one of his patients, he gives me a call. That day, although he wasn't sure, Jeremy thought he might be dealing with a genetic problem. During that phone call he told me the first part of the Moores' story.

MELISSA WAS THE first child born to Barry and Lisa. After an uncomplicated pregnancy and a picture-perfect delivery, the couple had taken the infant home to their townhouse in northern New Jersey. Lisa, who was 23 and had worked as a teacher's aide at a local nursery school, was on maternity leave from her job. Following three days of paternity leave, Barry, who was 25, resumed his daily commute into Manhattan, where he worked as a broker on Wall Street.

Within a week of the infant's arrival at home, the family's routine had become fairly well established. Melissa, at least during the first two weeks of her life, seemed like an ideal baby. A good eater with a strong suck, she was never fussy, crying only when she was hungry. Because Melissa was nursing, Lisa devoted most of her time to the baby's care; she'd nurse her, change her diaper, then rock her to sleep. Although during the first few nights Barry awoke with his wife for the two or three nocturnal feedings Melissa demanded, once he returned to work, he tended to sleep through the feedings. All in all, all three Moores seemed happy with their new lives.

But this peaceful existence lasted for less than two weeks.

On the morning of Melissa's 13th day of life, Lisa noticed that the child was crying. As I've already mentioned, Melissa usually cried only when she was hungry. But this wailing was different: although Lisa lifted Melissa out of her bassinet and prepared to nurse her, the baby refused to latch on to her mother's breast. Instead, she continued to scream at the top of her lungs.

Figuring the infant might be uncomfortable because of a wet diaper, Lisa began to undress her daughter. It was when she was removing Melissa's stretchy that Lisa noticed that the infant was holding her left arm limply at her side. Although her other arm and both legs were flailing, the left arm just hung there, flaccid. It was as if the arm had ceased to be a part of the baby.

Unsure of exactly what to do, Lisa called her mother. Hearing the sound of the baby crying in the background, Lisa's mother told her daughter to take the infant to the local emergency room immediately. Lisa re-dressed the still-screaming baby, put on her winter coat, snapped her into her car seat, and drove to the hospital. It was in the ER that the family's nightmare began.

MELISSA WAS SEEN almost immediately by one of the ER doctors. After asking only a few questions and briefly examining the infant, he sent the baby for an X-ray. Melissa was taken into one of the X-ray rooms by a technician, while Lisa was told to take a seat in the waiting area just outside.

According to Lisa, an inordinately long amount of time passed. Sitting alone in the nearly deserted waiting area, having not been separated from her daughter for more than a few minutes in the two weeks since Melissa had been born, Lisa said she felt as if one of her own arms had been amputated. After what seemed like hours, the ER doctor finally reappeared. He was accompanied by a woman who looked to be about 50. They took seats in the empty waiting area across from Lisa.

The woman, who said her name was Natalie Compton, did most of the talking. Very formally, she explained that she was the social worker assigned to the emergency room. She told Lisa that the X-rays that had been done on Melissa's left arm revealed that the infant had a fracture of the humerus, the bone that forms the upper portion of the arm. "Did the baby suffer any injuries in the past few hours?" Ms. Compton asked.

Lisa was shocked to hear that her daughter had a broken bone. With tears forming in her eyes and with a sudden urge to find her daughter and scoop her up into her arms, Lisa replied that no, Melissa had been in her bassinet sleeping peacefully prior to the time she started crying.

"Has anyone else been around the baby today?" Ms. Compton asked.

Lisa again responded no, that she and Melissa had been alone in the apartment since her husband had left for work early that morning. Ms. Compton asked for Barry's full name and his work number. After giving the social worker the information she requested, Lisa asked if she could see the baby.

"I'm afraid that won't be possible," Ms. Compton replied. "Because there isn't a good explanation for how the baby was injured, it is our legal responsibility to assume that Melissa is the victim of child abuse. As such, we will not be able to return the child to your care until a full investigation has been conducted and you and your husband have been cleared and are no longer considered suspects."

Shocked, Lisa rose to her feet. "Suspects?" she echoed. "You think I hurt my baby? You think I broke my baby's arm? Who do you think you are . . . ?" As Lisa lunged for the social worker, two hospital guards appeared, as if from out of the air. After intercepting her, they led Lisa to a small private room off the ER's main waiting room. While Lisa sat inside, alone, enraged, hurt, frightened, and sad, the guards kept vigil at the door.

The next few hours remain a blur in Lisa's mind. At some point a pair of local detectives entered the room to take a statement from Lisa; at another point a worker from the New Jersey Division of Youth and Family Services (DYFS) came in, introduced herself, and began the preliminary work needed to start an investigation; finally, Barry, who had been called by Ms. Compton at his office, appeared. Shaken but still functional, he led his now emotionally spent wife out of the hospital, across the parking lot, and to the car she had driven to the hospital hours before. Barry took Lisa home and put her to bed.

As the days passed, the nightmare intensified. A skeletal survey (X-rays of all the body's bones) revealed that in addition to the fracture of her left humerus, Melissa had three "old" broken ribs (fractures that had occurred some time in the recent past and now appeared to be in the process of healing). The investigation carried out by the DYFS worker failed to identify any cause for Melissa's broken bones. It was therefore assumed that the infant had been abused, beaten by either her mother or her father. The child, who had left the hospital in the care of an emergency foster parent, was placed in permanent foster care.

The Moores, who, according to the stipulations of the court order DYFS had obtained, were allowed to see their daughter only one hour a week during supervised visits, were advised by the attorney they retained that the only chance they had of ever getting Melissa back was if one of them pleaded guilty to the charges. "If neither of you accepts responsibility for this, there can never be any resolution," the attorney told them. "If one of you admits to having caused the fractures and enters into a course of therapy, a psychologist will eventually be able to report that it's safe to return Melissa to your care. Then there's a good chance they'll let you have her back."

After discussing it, although it seemed too bizarre to make sense, Barry and Lisa decided to take the advice: although she continued in private to maintain her innocence, Lisa admitted publicly to having beaten her child.

And that wasn't the end of it. Although the timing of Melissa's broken arm pointed to Lisa as the culprit, her broken ribs raised the possibility that Barry could have caused the injuries as well. Therefore, Lisa, who knew that she hadn't done anything to harm her daughter, blamed the rib injuries on her husband; Barry meanwhile, knowing full well that he was innocent, pointed to his wife as the perpetrator of the abuse. After fighting bitterly in the weeks following Melissa's visit to the ER, Barry took the inevitable step: unable to live with his presumed child-beating wife anymore, he moved out of the townhouse into a friend's apartment; he also retained an attorney for his own defense.

Lisa became progressively more depressed in the weeks following Barry's departure. The guilty plea colored every facet of her life. Her relationship with her husband was destroyed. She lost her job at the nursery school. Her friends stopped calling and coming by. Isolated and sad, she had trouble getting out of bed in the morning; she couldn't sleep and had no appetite. She began to have doubts: she'd do anything to get her daughter back, but admitting that she'd beaten Melissa may have been too much. Trying to find an answer, Lisa began reading everything she could find about child abuse. It was during that research that she stumbled upon the term *osteogenesis imperfecta,* a condition also known as brittle bone disease. Through her reading, Lisa became convinced that this disorder was the cause of Melissa's fractures. She called her pediatrician, Jeremy Stanger, to ask if Melissa could be tested for the disorder. It was that question that triggered Jeremy's initial telephone call to me.

OSTEOGENESIS IMPERFECTA (OI) is a relatively rare disease in which the bones are more fragile than normal. Caused by a mutation in one of the two genes responsible for the production of type I collagen, a protein that's an important building block of bones and connective tissue, OI is an inherited condition, often transmitted to the child from a parent who also has brittle bones. Individuals with OI show a wide range of severity. At its most severe, in the form of the disease called OI type II, the condition causes death in the newborn, whose skeleton is so fragile that the simple act of delivery causes every bone in the baby's body to fracture. Mercifully, most infants with this form of the disease are stillborn; however, I've unfortunately watched a few affected infants die due to respiratory failure, their ribs so shattered that the movements of the chest wall that result from the simple acts of inhaling and exhaling cause intense, unbearable pain. (In these rare cases, we are forced to provide so much narcotic pain medication to keep the babies comfortable that we depress the drive to breathe, hastening their death due to respiratory failure.) At its least severe, in OI type I, the individual may suffer one or two fractures during childhood, a number that wouldn't necessarily raise suspicion that anything was wrong. Most cases fall somewhere between these two extremes, with fractures occurring relatively often, usually resulting from incidents such as having a book bag fall on a foot or from being hit on the forearm with an errant basketball, events that would usually cause nothing more than a superficial bruise.

Although OI is a genetic disorder, in more than half of all cases, the family history is negative. In these children, as in the case in A.C. Sheridan, the change in the gene responsible for the condition arises spontaneously, through a new mutation in the genetic material. Although such individuals do not have parents who are affected, they can have affected children: regardless of how the mutation comes to be present, whether it be through inheritance or spontaneous change, each offspring born to an individual with OI has a 50 percent chance of also being affected.

When he called, Jeremy Stanger told me he had met the Moores on four occasions prior to the incident in the emergency room. "I know you can never be sure about these things," he said, "but these people did not strike me as child abusers. When the kid turned up with these fractures, I myself had trouble believing it. So when the mom called today, I realized she might be right. Is it possible this baby could have OI?"

I told him it was certainly possible, then added, "Unfortunately, most of the time in cases like this, it does turn out that one of the parents has been beating the child. But I've been involved in other cases in which kids have wound up in foster care because the diagnosis was missed. It's a real tragedy when it happens. Do you know if the X-rays were read by a pediatric radiologist?"

He told me the initial X-rays had been read by a radiologist in the emergency room who had not received any special training in pediatrics. "The X-ray findings in OI aren't subtle," he said. "The bones look washed out, different from a normal child's, with less calcium and thinner cortices, but it might not be something a general radiologist would pick up. The first step is to have the films reread by a pediatric radiologist." Then he asked, "Is that enough to prove the diagnosis?"

"It is to me," I said, "but since you've got the entire New Jersey criminal justice system involved here, it's probably going to be necessary to prove the diagnosis at the biochemical or molecular level. The only way to do that is to get a skin biopsy on the child and see if the collagen that her cells make is abnormal."

Jeremy transmitted this message to Lisa, whose attorney promptly petitioned the court to allow Melissa to undergo a skin biopsy, a minor surgical procedure. Although the paperwork dragged on for weeks, the judge who presided over the case finally granted approval when Melissa was a little over seven months old. The next day, the child was brought to the dermatologist who had consented to perform the procedure, and the sample of tissue was sent off by overnight express delivery to the lab in Seattle that does the testing for OI.

It took four months for the laboratory to finish its evaluation of Melissa's skin cells. Not surprisingly, when the final report was issued, it stated that Melissa's cells produced an abnormal form of type I procollagen, the precursor of type I collagen. The lab concluded that, as a result of this abnormality, the child from whom the sample had been obtained was affected with osteogenesis imperfecta type IV, a type of the disease that was somewhere between the severest form and the mildest form.

Melissa was nearly a year old when the social worker who was serving as her court-appointed guardian received the report from the lab. From that moment, the wheels of justice moved swiftly: within two days, a hearing was held and the judge ruled that, as a result of this new information, the child should be immediately returned to the care of her mother. Melissa was taken out of the foster home in which she'd lived for the past 11 months and moved back to the home of her mother, a relative stranger in this little girl's universe.

The family's visit to my office occurred a little more than a week after Melissa and her mother had been reunited. Although one would expect a child who'd been ripped out of the only home she'd known to have trouble adjusting to a new life, Melissa appeared to be fine. While her parents and I discussed OI and the problems she might have to face in the future, the little girl continued to play contentedly with her toys. I described the variable nature of the condition: "Although Melissa had a pretty rocky course in the first weeks of life, that doesn't necessarily mean she's going to have a lot of fractures in the future. I've seen kids who've had multiple fractures at birth continue to fracture during the first few months of life and then never suffer a fracture again. On the other hand, I've also seen kids who've had no fractures for the first year or two and who then begin to get them at the rate of six or seven per year. Where Melissa will fall in this range, I don't think any of us can predict."

"Isn't it strange that she had those four fractures while she was living with us and none for the entire year she was in foster care?" her father asked. From his accusatory tone, I got the feeling he was still trying to pin something on his ex-wife.

"It is a little strange, but it's not unheard of. Besides, we don't really know for sure if she's had any additional fractures or not. It's possible she's had some breaks that haven't been diagnosed. That's also something that's not unusual in children with OI. The only way to be sure is to do a skeletal survey." (Following our session, we did perform a skeletal survey, which showed that Melissa had in fact suffered two "silent" compression fractures of the spine while she had been in foster care. Our pediatric radiologist who read those films felt that these fractures could not have been caused by trauma.)

"Should Melissa's condition have been diagnosed in the emergency room?" her mother asked.

I hesitated. Before the family had come that day, I'd gotten copies of the original X-rays that had been done in the ER and reviewed them with our hospital's pediatric radiologist. Without any clinical information from me except for the age of the patient, he had looked at the films and said, "There's widespread osteopenia, and the skull shows obvious wormian bones. This is a child with osteogenesis imperfecta."

"Yes," I finally said. "Had the X-rays been read by a specialist in pediatric radiology, I think they would have been able to make the diagnosis back then."

"Then all of this would have been avoided," Lisa said sadly.

I didn't respond, but this mother knew that I agreed.

IT'S BEEN THREE MONTHS since the Moores first came to my office. Since then, Melissa has suffered no new fractures. Emotionally, she and her parents seem to be doing as well as can be expected, and a fragile bond has grown between the child and her mother, who has been granted custody (the father has weekend visitation rights). Although no one can predict what Melissa's future will be like, I have a good feeling that each member of the family will make it through this in reasonably good shape.

In the time that's passed since I first met them, I've thought repeatedly about the tragedy the Moore family has had to endure. Needlessly, this child was separated from her parents during the most critical year of her life. Her parents, having come to mistrust and disbelieve each other, split apart, with apparently no possibility of reconciliation. The mother lost her job, her friends, and ultimately her dignity. All of this because a diagnosis that should have been made in an ER went unmade.

In retrospect, this *was* a case of abuse. It wasn't abuse inflicted by a parent on a child; rather, it was abuse inflicted on an innocent family by an overzealous system.

Postscript

IT'S NOW BEEN ten years since Melissa was taken away from her mother in the emergency room of a hospital in northern New Jersey. Her parents, still not what you'd consider the best of friends, are now at least civil to each other. Having realized that their suspicions about each other's role in causing their daughter's fractures were unfounded, they were able to forgive each other; however, the anger and hostility that grew between them during the time after Melissa was removed from their custody will forever prevent them from becoming friends. As Melissa's mother has said to me on more than one occasion, "There's some water that just won't pass under the bridge."

Both parents have remarried, and Melissa's father has gone on to have two more children. As of now, Lisa has not had the nerve to have another baby. Although I've told her that, because studies of the parents' DNA revealed that Melissa's mutation in *COL1A1* (one of two genes responsible for the formation of type 1 collagen) arose spontaneously and that the risk of recurrence of OI in a subsequent child is less than 1 percent, I have the feeling that she just doesn't believe me. But after what she went through, I'm not sure anyone would blame her.

Since Melissa's birth, we've seen great strides in the treatment of the more severe forms of OI, or at least in those severely affected children who survive the newborn period. In a landmark paper published in the *New England Journal of Medicine* in 1998, Francis H. Glorieux and his colleagues in Montreal reported on their success in treating children with severe OI with pamidronate, a drug that, like the more commonly used

Fosamax (alendronate sodium) is a bisphosphonate, a class of medications that inhibit the rate at which bone is resorbed.[1] (Although they look like static, stable structures, bones are actually extremely dynamic; they are constantly being broken down and rebuilt; the rate of resorption of old bone and reconstruction of new bone is under strict genetic control.) After giving the medication for approximately one year, the Montreal group was able to demonstrate improved bone density in children with the severe forms of OI, which led to a markedly decreased number of fractures, which in turn led to improved ambulatory function in children with OI. As a result of this study and others that followed, treatment with pamidronate has become a standard part of the care we provide for children and adults with forms of OI that are at the more severe end of the spectrum.

But Melissa, who had so many fractures in the first two weeks of her life, never became a candidate for pamidronate therapy. Amazingly, since being returned to her mother's custody, she has suffered not a single additional fracture. As I said when I spoke with the family in the days after the diagnosis was confirmed, I've seen this happen in patients. OI is a tricky disease. Some people will have many fractures evenly spaced from birth until puberty. (The condition usually becomes quiescent after puberty, due to the stabilizing effect that testosterone and estrogen have on bone density; in women, bone fragility returns after menopause, but in affected men few fractures ever recur.) Others, like Melissa, will have many fractures early in life but far fewer after the first year or two. Still others will not fracture at all until after their second birthday and then will have dozens of fractures. There seems to be no rhyme or reason for why this happens, no great correlation between the genotype (that is, where in the *COL1A1* or *COL1A2* genes the mutation occurs) and the phenotype (i.e., the actual expression of the disease in the individual) that would allow us to predict the course of one individual's disease.

Melissa has also grown extremely well; as compared with other kids with OI, whose growth is stunted by the abnormality in their type I collagen, Melissa's height has been excellent, consistently between the 50th and 75th percentiles on the growth curve. It's a little weird: although her early history of multiple fractures, along with the DNA and biochemical studies that were done on her skin biopsy cells, tells us that she definitely has OI type IV, to see her now, to review her history since she returned home to live with her mother, it's as if she has been cured. Of course, that's not the case; we'll have to follow her very closely as she ages. But for now I expect that she'll live a full and healthy life.

Melissa's case spotlights another role played by clinical geneticists. Often called on to solve mysteries, we play the role of medical detective, noticing subtle symptoms and signs and assembling them into a cohesive diagnosis. One of the heroes of modern clinical geneticists is Sherlock Holmes, Sir Arthur Conan Doyle's amazing detective. It was in Doyle's story "A Case of Identity" that Holmes says, "It is my business to know things. Perhaps I have taught myself to see what others overlook." This is exactly the mantra of the clinical geneticist.

One could argue that had the emergency room doctors sought a genetics consultation before calling DYFS, the misery that occurred in Melissa's first year of life could have been averted. In my opinion, we geneticists are underutilized in this role. Employing us to help solve medical puzzles can be helpful to both colleagues in other medical specialties and, more important, to families like the Moores, in which the solution might have prevented their child from winding up in foster care. Thus, our ability to solve puzzles can sometimes be a blessing; at other times, however, it can be a curse.

CHAPTER 3

The Reunion

W HEN I GOT the letter in the mail, my initial inclination was to throw it in the trash and forget I'd ever received it. I mean, after nearly two decades of being out of contact with all the people with whom I'd shared those years, I looked forward to attending my 20th-year college reunion with about as much glee as I do to undergoing a root canal. After tearing open the envelope and reading its contents, I dropped the letter onto the pile of papers on my desk without giving it so much as a second thought.

But then, a few days later, out of the clear blue, I got a call from Andy Bennett, my old roommate. "Did you get the invitation?" he asked.

"Yeah," I replied. "I was absolutely thrilled."

"I think Debbie and I might bring our kids out for it," he said.

"Andy, are you telling me you're seriously considering spending a couple thousand dollars in airfare and wasting half a day traveling in each direction in order to return to the Armpit of New England?" I used the term Andy and I had submitted during our junior year when the Worcester Chamber of Commerce, during an ill-conceived campaign to improve the city's image, had sponsored a contest to find the perfect nickname for the city. (Our entry, by the way, did not win.)

"Well, when you put it that way, Bob, maybe we ought to reconsider," he replied. But then he explained that he and his wife had been looking for an excuse to bring their kids east to show them some of the places he'd lived when he was young, and as it turned out, the timing of the reunion fit their schedule perfectly. "If we come, would you consider joining us?" he finally asked.

I promised that if he and his family were willing to fly all the way out to Massachusetts, my family and I would be waiting in the lobby of the majestic and stately Worcester Holiday Inn to greet them.

ANDY AND I had been roommates during the last three years of college. We'd made our home a few blocks off campus in a remarkably sleazy apartment located on the second floor of a run-down triple-decker (a form of architecture apparently unique to that region of New England). In addition to sharing that apartment and all the responsibilities that came with living on our own, we'd become close friends, coming to depend on each other for support during that terrible first semester of our senior year, when Andy received a series of rejections from law schools and I received a similar series from medical schools.

We'd both managed to get in somewhere, though, and after graduation Andy went off to Chicago, where he met and married Debbie, while I landed at the Royal College of Surgeons in Dublin, Ireland. After finishing law school, Andy and Debbie ultimately settled in Seattle, where Andy joined a large law firm. Meanwhile, after only a year in Ireland, I'd managed to get accepted at Einstein in New York, and my wife, Beth, and I had put down roots in the Northeast. For the first few years, we'd all managed to stay in touch by phone and mail. But then, about 12 years before, life had become a little too hectic and we'd lost contact. Unfortunately, Beth and I hadn't communicated with the Bennetts until the reunion letter came in the mail.

AS IT TURNED OUT, when Beth and I arrived in the lobby of the Worcester Holiday Inn, it was the Bennetts who were there waiting for us. Our monthly spina bifida clinic was held that Friday afternoon, and as a result I couldn't leave the hospital until after five o'clock. By the time I'd arrived home, packed up the car, corralled the kids, and headed for the highway, it had already been nearly seven. We didn't make it to the hotel until a little after ten.

By then, Andy and Debbie had already put their kids to sleep. After we checked in, the Bennetts accompanied us to our rooms, and while Beth was getting our kids into bed, Debbie, Andy, and I tried to fill in some of the blanks. Their lives seemed almost storybook perfect: at his law firm, Andy had made partner a few years before and was now pulling in the big bucks; Debbie, who had trained as an elementary school teacher, had taken a leave of absence from her job and was spending her time raising their two children. They lived in a gorgeous house on an acre of land that had a magnificent view of Puget Sound.

Their lives seemed wonderful except for one possible flaw: it appeared that there was some trouble with the Bennetts' younger child, Rebecca, and the couple was having difficulty coming to grips with it. Debbie explained that the little girl, who was then three and a half, seemed to be developing at a much slower rate than had Eric, the couple's ten-year-old. Rebecca hadn't begun walking until 20 months, and even now she seemed clumsy and poorly coordinated; she hadn't said any words until she was nearly two, and at this point she still hadn't begun to put two-word phrases together.

But when Debbie began explaining how worried she was about her younger child, Andy cut her off: "There's really nothing wrong with her," he explained to Beth and me with a forced smile on his face. "She just happens to be a slow starter. That's what our doctor told us, isn't it, Deb?" His wife only looked away, and my old roommate went on: "Our pediatrician gave her a complete examination and did some blood work, and he told us he couldn't find anything wrong with her. He said he was positive she was fine, and he was sure she would catch up with time." And then to his wife he added, "I don't understand why you always have to be so pessimistic about everything."

The conflict between Andy and Debbie seemed to take the steam out of our conversation. Although the Bennetts were still on West Coast time, it was nearly midnight in Worcester, and Beth and I were exhausted. Saturday was going to be a big day: there was a barbecue on campus for all alumni and their families at noon, an afternoon filled with tours and activities, and an evening reception back at the hotel. We promised to meet in the lobby at about eleven o'clock in the morning.

I KNEW THERE was something wrong with Rebecca the moment I laid eyes on her in the hotel's lobby. She looked different from the rest of her family, much heavier than either her brother or her parents, and her eyes had a vacant look. I tried to talk with her, tried to engage her in a silly conversation, but she wouldn't respond, choosing instead to hide behind her mother's denim skirt. "Don't be afraid," Debbie said gently, placing her arm around the girl's shoulder. "This is our friend Bob. He's a nice man." But no matter how reassuring her parents were, Rebecca wouldn't come forward.

On the ride over to campus, packed into Beth's station wagon, I surreptitiously tried to gather information. Andy mentioned in passing that Rebecca had a tremendous appetite, that she was able to eat far more than her older brother; Debbie said that both Rebecca and Eric were in excellent health, never sick a day. "In fact, the only time either of my kids spent any time in the hospital was the day Rebecca had surgery to remove her extra fingers when she was a baby," she stated matter-of-factly.

"She was born with extra fingers?" I asked, understanding immediately the significance of this announcement.

"Mm-hmm," Andy replied. "Extra toes, too. Debbie was the one who picked it up in the delivery room. 'Aren't babies only supposed to have 20 fingers and toes?' she asked our obstetrician. Can you imagine? Everyone else missed it."

So as not to arouse suspicion, I steered the discussion away from Rebecca at that point. But the information I'd been given was enough for me: there was clearly something wrong with this little girl. Now all I had to do was figure out what to do with this information.

SUCH DILEMMAS ARE an inevitable consequence of being a clinical geneticist. During my training, I was taught to search for subtle, seemingly disparate problems—conditions such as obesity and polydactyly (having too many fingers and toes) and developmental delay—and assemble them, like the pieces of a jigsaw puzzle, into a single unifying picture. And because of my training, because of the way clinical geneticists are taught to approach problems, wherever I go, whomever I see, regardless of the setting, I can't help but observe features, note anomalies, compile lists, and make diagnoses.

Outside my office, what happens once those diagnoses are made creates the dilemma. Clinical genetics is unique: unlike other medical specialties, the implications of a diagnosis extend beyond the individual affected with the disease. Because of the inherited nature of many of these conditions, because of the fact that they're often passed from parent to child, detection and disclosure of a genetic diagnosis have consequences not only for the patient but also for his or her children, siblings, parents, and other family members. So when a geneticist feels strongly that the three-year-old walking with his father through Kmart has Williams syndrome (a disorder caused by a deletion of a small portion of chromosome 7), or the guy sitting in front of him at Yankee Stadium has Treacher

Collins syndrome (an inherited condition that causes conductive hearing loss and facial malformations), or a pediatric resident has myotonic dystrophy (a form of muscular dystrophy that's passed down from parent to child), or the daughter of his college roommate has Bardet-Biedl syndrome, what is he to do? What is my legal responsibility? And more important, what is my ethical responsibility?

Unfortunately, I haven't been able to answer these questions to my own satisfaction. In fact, I chose not to say anything to either the parents of the child in Kmart or the guy at Yankee Stadium; I did manage to have a conversation with the pediatric resident and suggested that she go to see a neurologist, but I failed to mention that the cause for my concern was that she might have myotonic dystrophy. But my dilemma intensified that day in Worcester as I turned over in my head the risks and benefits of telling my old friend, who was clearly deep in denial, that his only daughter might very well be affected with a disease that not only had caused her to have obesity, polydactyly, and developmental delay but also, with the passage of time, would cause her to lose her vision (due to pigmentary retinopathy, a condition that causes progressive degeneration of vision) and possibly develop renal failure, and that, because of its inherited nature, could recur in future children. Late that afternoon, after nearly four hours of having the internal argument of whether to speak up or not rage in my head, I finally came to a decision.

While the afternoon festivities were beginning to wind down, I asked Debbie if she would come for a walk with me. As we walked away from the greensward that had served as the site for most of the afternoon's activities, I explained to her my concern that Rebecca had Bardet-Biedl syndrome. "I can't be a hundred percent sure," I told her, "but the obesity, polydactyly, and developmental delay are all there. At the very least, she needs to have her eyes examined and her kidneys checked."

Rather than becoming distraught at this news, Debbie seemed almost relieved. I wasn't surprised by this: having already come to the conclusion that something was wrong with her daughter, she was almost happy to find out that she wasn't crazy, as her husband and their pediatrician had suggested. But her relief proved to be short-lived: when I finally told her about the long-term problems associated with the disorder, she became tearful. We were silent for a while as she composed herself again. Then she said, "What do we do about Andy?"

After more hesitation I finally answered, "I guess I'll have a talk with him."

IT WAS AFTER MIDNIGHT. The main event, the reception for our class that had been held in the main ballroom of the Holiday Inn, had ended. Andy and I were sitting alone in the hotel's bar, drinking beer and calmly reminiscing about the deep, dark past. It was getting late; I knew I couldn't put off this difficult job much longer. Finally, I just leaped into it. "Andy," I said, "I'm a little concerned about Rebecca."

"What?" my friend asked, obviously confused by this complete non sequitur.

"I think Debbie's feelings about her are right. She does seem to have some problems. I think she may have a condition called Bardet-Biedl syndrome. People with Bardet-Biedl have polydactyly, developmental delay, obesity, and visual problems. She needs to have some tests done, but—"

"What are you talking about?" Andy nearly shouted, his calm demeanor instantly vanishing. "She's fine. Our pediatrician went over her with a fine-tooth comb. He told us there was nothing wrong with her."

"It's not a common condition," I replied. "It's not something a general pediatrician would be expected to know about."

"Oh, so you think you know more than our pediatrician, huh? You, my college roommate who couldn't even get into an American medical school? You spend a couple of minutes with my daughter and you think you know more about her than the doctor who's been seeing her and following her since she was a baby?" Andy, now raging, had risen to his feet by this point. "You know what? You should learn to mind your own business!" And with that, he turned and stormed out of the bar.

BY THE TIME we came down for breakfast the next morning, the Bennetts were gone. They had checked out of their room, I guessed, and moved on to the rest of their tour of places Andy had lived when he was growing up. It's been four months since the reunion weekend ended; we haven't heard a word from them.

Since returning home from Worcester, I've spent a lot of time wondering whether handling the situation in a different way might have produced a better outcome. Perhaps I should have asked Debbie for the name and telephone number of Rebecca's pediatrician and spoken directly with the doctor, apprising him of my concern. Maybe I should have sent Debbie a packet of information about Bardet-Biedl syndrome in the mail and let her deal with the situation herself. Or maybe I should have done exactly as Andy had suggested: just minded my own business. I don't know if any of these would have resulted in a different response from my old roommate.

I've come to realize that there's no wrong or right answer to any of this. There are only frustration and anger and, unfortunately, the apparent loss of an old friend.

Postscript

SINCE OUR REUNION WEEKEND, I've neither seen nor heard from either Andy or Debbie Bennett. I don't know if their daughter turned out to have Bardet-Biedl syndrome; I don't know if they've gone on to have other kids who might have also been affected with this condition. (Bardet-Biedl syndrome is inherited in an autosomal recessive manner, meaning that in order to have it, a child needs to inherit one copy of a nonworking gene from each parent. Such parents, who are carriers, are physically normal; however, each child born to such parents has a one-in-four chance of also being affected.) It's sad that our relationship ended that way, but I did what I thought was right, and I'm now forced to live with the consequences.

Even after all these years, I've still never really figured out what I should do when placed in the situation I was in with Rebecca Bennett. Being able to make a diagnosis simply by looking at a face continues to be both a blessing and a curse, especially when the condition carries with it serious consequences for the individual.

Here's an example, a problem that's been haunting me for the past few years: On News 12 Westchester, the local TV station carried by our cable system, the weatherman, a seemingly very nice guy, clearly has the facial features of Crouzon syndrome. An inherited condition similar to (though much milder than) Pfeiffer syndrome, the disease that affects A.C. Sheridan, Crouzon syndrome combines an unusual facial appearance and premature closure of the sutures of the skull. The premature closure can lead to increased pressure within the skull, which can result in herniation of the brain stem through the foramen magnum, the opening in the back of the skull that allows the spinal cord and the brain to connect.

Herniation of the brain stem can result in sudden death. This might be what happened to Marty Feldman, the actor best remembered for his portrayal of Igor (or Eye-gor) in Mel Brooks's *Young Frankenstein*. Feldman, who had the typical facial appearance, including the proptotic eyes, of an individual with Crouzon syndrome, died suddenly in his sleep at the age of 48. I believe that Feldman's death was a consequence of the increased intracranial pressure caused by herniation of his brainstem, an event that was directly related to his underlying disease.

With my knowledge of both Marty Feldman's fate and the reaction of my old roommate, what am I to do about my impression that the News 12 weatherman, someone I've never even met, is also affected with this disorder and therefore possibly at risk? Should I call him and tell him of my concerns? Should I e-mail or write him? Should I just assume that because he's lived in the New York metropolitan area for all these years, he would have already consulted a physician and received a diagnosis? Or should I take Andy's instructions and just mind my own business?

I have to admit that, for good or for bad, my experience with the Bennetts has colored my reaction to this dilemma: in the case of the News 12 weatherman, I decided to keep the information to myself. But every night I make sure to watch the local news, and not because I'm so interested in the activities of our community: I'm just making sure that the weatherman is still alive!

CHAPTER 4

Scotty's Funeral

I CIRCLED THE FUNERAL home three times before finally turning into the driveway. "Why the hell are you doing this?" I kept asking myself out loud. "You don't belong here! You barely know these people!" I had, I argued in rebuttal to each of these points, promised the Thompsons that I'd be at the funeral. So, reluctantly, after finally convincing myself to commit, I approached the driveway one last time, made a right turn, and looked for a place to park.

It was the Saturday of what had been a bad week. The previous Sunday, one of my patients, an infant with a rare form of dwarfism called Jarcho-Levin syndrome, had died in the neonatal intensive care unit. After two weeks of life, her lungs, smaller than normal because of the abnormalities of the bones that formed her chest, had finally failed, and in spite of the fact that she'd been attached to a ventilator since birth, she suffocated. Her death was frustrating because there was absolutely nothing any of us could do to help her even though we knew exactly what was wrong.

Then, on Monday afternoon, in the nursery at University Hospital, I examined a newborn who had features of Down syndrome and went to talk to her parents. After long and frustrating meetings both that day and the next, the parents decided to place their baby in foster care. These sessions affected me badly. Because I'd failed as an advocate for the baby, I felt as if I'd let him down; at the same time, by introducing my own feelings into the counseling sessions, by telling the parents what I thought they should do rather than listening to what they wanted to do, I hadn't been able to serve as an effective counselor during their time of need.

And during the course of the week, while all this had been happening, a number of my other patients became sick. Two of the children I follow in the spina bifida clinic developed infections of their ventriculoperitoneal shunts (the plastic tubes that connect the ventricle of the brain to the peritoneal cavity of the abdomen, designed to treat hydrocephalus by draining the excess fluid that collects around the brain), and in spite of megadoses of antibiotics, neither infection seemed to want to clear. And on Tuesday, a boy with Down syndrome, a child to whom I'd grown attached since his birth months before, came into my office for a regular visit covered with petechiae, red blotches on his skin; evaluation over the next two days showed that he had acute megakaryocytic leukemia, a rare hematologic malignancy with a poor prognosis. As a result of all this, I'd come home from work Thursday hopeless and demoralized, doubting I was doing anybody any good, thinking seriously for the first time in years about the possibility of a career change.

And then, at a little after ten o'clock that evening, when the few hours of separation from my office had allowed my spirits to lift a little, the phone rang. It was Steve Thompson. His son, Scotty, he told me, had been declared dead in the emergency room at Bronxville Hospital a few hours earlier. "It happened the way you said it would," he told me, trying to hold back tears. "He just stopped breathing. By the time we got him to the ER, he was gone."

Like the death of my patient with Jarcho-Levin syndrome, this was not unexpected news; Scotty Thompson had trisomy 13, a chromosome abnormality that is lethal during the first year of life in 90 percent of affected infants.

"How's Nancy?" I asked.

"Pretty broken up. We're both pretty broken up. We just wanted to let you know."

I sighed. "I'm sorry, Steve," I said. "I wish there was something I could say that would make this all better. I guess, all things considered, it's for the best."

Steve agreed, but added, "That doesn't make it any easier."

We said goodbye, and I spent the rest of the night thinking about the Thompsons and all that had happened to them since we'd first met in the neonatal intensive care unit at University Hospital five weeks before.

I'D BEEN GETTING ready to leave that Thursday afternoon when my office phone rang. It was Dr. Laura Kenyon, the neonatologist in charge of University Hospital's NICU. She explained that an infant with multiple congenital anomalies had just been transferred from Bronxville Hospital. "He's having respiratory distress. Sometime tonight, I'm probably going to have to make a decision about whether to intubate him and put him on a ventilator. I wouldn't want to do that if I know he has something lethal."

Understanding from the tone of Laura's voice that this was one of those rare genetic emergencies, I told her I was already on my way over.

Meeting me at the unit's door and handing me a sterile gown, Laura began telling me the story in NICU-ese: "It's an SGA full-termer, born five hours ago to a 32-year-old primigravida at Bronxville." To translate: He was a full-term baby but small for his gestational age; this was his mother's first pregnancy. Laura continued, "He was sent to us because of congenital anomalies and respiratory distress." As she led me into one of the patient rooms, I pulled on the gown. "The prenatal course was unremarkable," Laura said. "After six hours of uneventful labor, this kid popped out."

We stopped at one of the room's warming tables and I laid eyes on Scotty Thompson for the first time. Three things about him were immediately clear: first, he was in severe respiratory distress, his hands and mouth blue because of lack of oxygen; second, as Laura had mentioned, he had some obvious congenital defects; and finally, apart from these two serious problems, the baby had a headful of the brightest red hair I'd ever seen.

I immediately set about examining him. Scotty had many unusual features. Thin and scrawny, he had microcephaly (an unusually small head), a sloping forehead, microphthalmia (eyes that were smaller than they should have been), a beaked nose, and low-set malformed ears. In addition, he had six fingers on each hand and six toes on each foot, a small penis, and testicles that had not yet descended into his small scrotum. The baby's overall appearance confirmed my initial impression. "He's got trisomy 13," I told Laura, who was standing next to me.

"Are you sure?" she asked. "Would you be willing to write that in the chart?"

I recognized the significance of Laura's question. To a neonatologist, confirmation from a geneticist that a baby has trisomy 13 means that nothing heroic should or would be done to prolong the baby's life. Because the prognosis for babies with this condition is so poor, my diagnosis would mean that Laura would not order Scotty to be placed on a ventilator if his breathing worsened; she would not force any surgical procedures on him, even if subsequent evaluation revealed a life-threatening internal malformation. That was a lot of responsibility to put in my hands, so I did what I usually do in cases like this: I hedged. "I'm pretty sure," I answered, knowing full well that being pretty sure just wouldn't be good enough for her. "You know the only way to be 100 percent sure is to do the chromosome analysis."

"Bob, chromosome studies will take at least a day," Laura responded. "I need to know tonight."

"Well, let me check one thing," I said softly. I knew there was one finding that was essentially pathognomonic (i.e., diagnostic) for trisomy 13. Cleaning the back of the baby's scalp with a saline-soaked gauze pad, I searched the skin.

I found them immediately just to the left of the occiput: two small punched-out lesions in the skin that had gone unnoticed because of the thick crop of red hair but that now virtually sealed this infant's fate. "Aplasia cutis congenita," I said to Laura. "Punched-out lesions of the scalp. That confirms the diagnosis. We'll do chromosomes anyway, but there's no question about it. This baby's definitely got trisomy 13."

I went to the nurses' station to write a note in the infant's chart. When I was about halfway through, the ward clerk told me that the baby's father had arrived and was waiting to speak to me in Laura Kenyon's office. Putting down the chart, I went to join him.

STEVE THOMPSON WAS sitting on the couch in Laura's office. He was terrified. After introducing myself, I sat on Laura's desk chair and asked how he was doing.

"Not well," he replied. He was about my age and seemed as if he'd been through the ringer; his clothes were wrinkled, his face was pale, and he looked as if he could use a good night's sleep. "They told us at the other hospital that the baby's got a lot of problems."

I nodded. "I think he has a condition called trisomy 13."

"What's that?" he asked without much change in his expression.

"It's a condition that's caused by the presence of an extra copy of a chromosome in every cell of the body. The extra chromosome causes all sorts of malformations, some of which we can see on the surface and some that are internal."

His eyes were beginning to cloud over with tears now. "What . . . what . . . ?" was all he could manage to get out.

I continued without allowing him to finish his question.

"Unfortunately, the baby's chances are not good," I went on mechanically, trying not to make eye contact as I was saying these words. "Almost all babies with trisomy 13 die before their first birthday, and most die within the first two or three months. Less than 10 percent survive past age one." I stopped there; the choked-off cries I was hearing from Mr. Thompson told me that I'd made my point and that going on would have been sadistic.

Tears were forming in my eyes as, waiting uncomfortably, I occasionally looked up into this man's face, seeing the pain he was feeling. Finally, controlling himself, he uttered, "You're sure?"

"No, not 100 percent sure," I replied. "We need to do a blood test to confirm it. But, Mr. Thompson, I have to tell you, I'm sure enough to be talking to you like this. If I wasn't fairly certain, I wouldn't be putting you through this torture."

He nodded. "I appreciate your honesty," he managed. "It means a lot to know that you're not keeping anything from me. Where do we go from here?"

"Well, Dr. Kenyon, the neonatologist, is going to want to talk to you. Because of his breathing problems, there's a good chance the baby might need to be put on a ventilator later tonight. She needs to know what your feelings are about that."

He stared blankly, so I continued: "A lot of times, when a baby has trisomy 13, the parents and doctors decide together that nothing heroic should be done to keep the infant going."

"I can't make any decisions without talking to my wife," he said.

"It makes things difficult, her being in another hospital," I responded. "It's got to be tough on both of you, having to go through this on your own, without having the other to lean on."

He nodded, and tears filled his eyes again.

"I'd be happy to talk with her on the phone," I added, "if you think it would help."

"No, I'll tell her."

"Do you have any questions?"

He sat silently for a few seconds, and then shook his head.

"I'm sorry we had to meet this way. I wish I could have brought you better news," I said, beginning to rise from my chair. "The next few weeks aren't going to be easy. You should always remember that Dr. Kenyon and I are here to help you guys through this. If you have any questions, or if you need to talk, give me a call anytime. That's what I'm here for."

He wiped away the tears as I brought him into the NICU to see his son. After helping him into a gown, I led him to Scotty's bedside. Upon seeing the red-haired boy, his eyes again filled with tears.

I left him there, staring at the baby. After telling Laura Kenyon about our discussion, I picked up my coat and briefcase and left the hospital, the image of Steve Thompson's grim face lined up next to the faces of all the other grim-faced mothers and fathers I'd left standing by their babies' bedsides over the years now a permanent part of my memory.

SCOTTY THOMPSON NEVER needed to be placed on a ventilator. Within hours of my visit, his respiratory distress resolved. To identify internal anomalies, Laura and I undertook a limited workup. We discovered that although his heart, intestines, and kidneys all seemed to be functioning normally, he had holo-prosencephaly, a severe developmental abnormality of the brain, which would certainly shorten his life. But in spite of this anomaly, he acted pretty much the way any infant should during those first few days: he took formula from a bottle, breathed on his own, and maintained his pulse and blood pressure without assistance. And on his third day of life, I received a preliminary report from our cytogenetics lab confirming the presence of an extra copy of chromosome 13 in every one of his cells that was examined.

When I came by on rounds on the afternoon of Scotty's second day, I found Mrs. Thompson sitting by her son's bedside. Holding the tiny baby in her arms, she was trying with difficulty to feed him from a bottle, while she sobbed softly. I introduced myself, and she told me that she and her husband had discussed the things I'd told him the day before; they had decided to ask Laura Kenyon to write a "do not resuscitate" order in the baby's chart. "We know he doesn't have much of a chance," she explained. "Neither Steve nor I want to put Scotty through anything painful. We want him to be as comfortable as possible."

On that first day, we talked mostly about practical issues; I answered a lot of the questions that had been left unanswered since her baby had been born. Were Scotty's problems possibly caused by anything she'd done during the pregnancy? (No, I told her, the baby's extra chromosome was present before he was even conceived in either the sperm or the egg that had formed him, and that nothing that had happened after conception could in any way have altered the eventual outcome.) Was the baby's problem in any way caused by her work? (She was a lawyer who had commuted by train from Westchester to Manhattan every day during the first trimester of pregnancy; I told her that, as far as we knew, riding Metro North had never been implicated as a cause of chromosomal abnormalities.) Should her obstetrician have done anything to detect Scotty's problems before he was born? (Although an amniocentesis would have detected the chromosome abnormality, Mrs. Thompson was not considered a high-risk patient, meaning that there was no reason to refer her for an amnio; further, for reasons that were not clear, a serum triple-screen test, a maternal blood test designed to identify pregnancies at increased risk for trisomies, had been totally normal.)

We talked for nearly an hour that day. I felt comfortable with her, as if we were old friends. Near the end of the time we spent together, she asked a question that had probably been on her mind all along, one she must have found very difficult to ask: "Where do we go from here?"

Her question caught me a little off guard. "What do you mean?" I asked.

"Well, Scotty seems okay to me. I understand he's got a lot of problems, but they're not doing anything for him here that I couldn't do at home. Do we take him home with us, or what?"

"There are basically two options," I replied carefully. This was tricky terrain; what to do with the infant from here on was a decision to be made solely by the Thompsons, not by me, Laura Kenyon, or any other physician involved in the baby's care. I needed to relay the information without coloring it in any way with my own personal bias. "You could either arrange to put him into placement or take him home with you," I explained succinctly.

"If we wanted him placed, how would that happen?" she asked. "Where would he go?"

I had my answer already prepared; I'd been thinking of this since the day I'd first seen the infant: "There are two options. We could arrange a foster care placement with a family in this area. Or there's a pediatric hospice in Queens that only takes children who have less than six months to live. It's a very nice place; if you'd like, I can get you information about it; if you want to go further, I can help arrange a visit."

"And what would taking him home mean?" she asked cautiously.

"Well, basically, it would mean that you and your husband would be providing all his care. We could arrange for some assistance from the visiting nurse service, but for the most part it would be you guys and Scotty."

"Do you think we could do that?" she asked, and I could tell by the tone of her voice and the look in her eyes that she wanted, maybe even needed, to take this baby home. "Neither of us has any nursing experience or anything like that. Do you think we could manage to take care of him ourselves?"

I nodded. "I definitely think you can."

"And what if we try and it doesn't work out?" she asked. "What if we get him home and find we just can't take care of him?"

"No decision's permanent," I replied. "If you've given it a try and find you can't manage, we can always place Scotty at that point."

That was when she smiled for the first time during that entire hour. I knew right then that her mind had been made up.

THE THOMPSONS TOOK Scotty home two days later, vowing that they would make whatever time he had on earth worthwhile. The baby's life wasn't easy: he slept all day and stayed awake all night screaming; he continued to suck reasonably well, but two days after discharge he began to vomit and seemed to develop a bad case of colic. Steve and Nancy stayed awake every night with Scotty, taking turns holding him, trying their best to comfort him, but each attempt met with failure. They spent their days like zombies, trying to conduct their lives as if nothing had changed. As I watched from a distance, I wondered how long they'd be able to hold on.

I talked with them, either by phone or in person, just about every weekday after Scotty's discharge; as is inevitable in cases like this, we grew closer with each passing contact. During the early days after the baby's discharge, we talked about many things, from the issue of whether his colic might be a sign of some undiagnosed intestinal malformation, to the risk for having a second child affected with trisomy 13 (the recurrence risk was 1 percent for every subsequent pregnancy). But, as time passed, our conversations evolved more and more to questions concerning the infant's eventual and nearly certain demise. "How will Scotty die?" Nancy called to ask one day when the infant was three weeks old.

I knew the question would come up sooner or later, and I was glad when it did. Talking about Scotty's death, asking concrete questions about the event, was a sure sign that Nancy was making progress in her mourning process.

"He'll probably die of apnea," I answered softly. "That is, he'll just stop breathing. We know his brain's not formed properly, and it's the brain that controls breathing. Most likely, you or Steve will find him lying in his crib one morning, and that will be it."

There was silence on the other end of the phone.

During Scotty's visit to my office when he was four weeks old, the Thompsons were upbeat, reporting that the child seemed to have turned a corner. The colic had resolved; he was no longer vomiting as much, and he didn't seem to be in any pain. And, much to the relief of his parents, he was now sleeping for three- and four-hour stretches during the night.

The Thompsons also appeared as if they had turned a corner that day. Steve looked better rested than he'd been at any time since I'd known him; there was a smile on his face as he held his son and pointed out that Scotty had not lost any of his bright red hair and, if anything, it was coming in thicker and redder than ever. And Nancy, too, looked good; I got the sense that they had come to the point of acceptance in the mourning process. It was at that moment I realized they were going to be okay.

I told them I was happy that things were going so well. But then I examined Scotty. And I realized that their sense of acceptance had not come a moment too soon.

During the course of my very brief physical examination, Scotty had an apnea spell: he completely stopped breathing for about 25 seconds; during this episode, his skin color changed from its natural pink, first to dusky blue, then to dark blue, and finally to deep gray. I was beginning to think about whether I should begin to resuscitate on him or whether just letting nature take its course was a better plan when, at last, he took a deep breath; within seconds, his color improved. Although he recovered this time, I knew it wasn't going to be long; I had seen a prelude to Scotty's death, and I knew it was time to get the Thompsons ready for it.

I didn't say a word to them during my exam, but after the baby was again dressed and we'd reassembled in my office, I told Steve and Nancy what I felt they needed to know. "Scotty had a long breath-holding spell while I was examining him," I said. "That's usually an important sign in kids with trisomy 13. I don't think he's got much longer."

They looked at me but didn't utter a word.

I continued, "As I told you, Nancy, I think he's going to simply stop breathing one day and that'll be it. Judging from the spell I saw, it could be anytime now."

The silence that followed lasted for at least a minute. The happy expressions that had been on their faces had melted away. "What . . . what should we do if . . . ?" Steve finally asked. "Should we call an ambulance? Should we call our pediatrician? Should we call you?"

And just then I did something I'd never done before: I essentially choreographed the death of one of my patients. "When you find him, you should call an ambulance. The paramedics will come, pick him up, and transport him to the hospital—"

"Will I be able to ride with him?" Nancy interrupted.

"Probably," I replied. "Although each ambulance corps has its own rules and regulations, I can't imagine that anyone would give you a hard time. Anyway, the ambulance will probably take him to the emergency room at Bronxville Hospital; he'll be seen by a physician there who'll declare him dead—"

"Should we try to resuscitate him?" Steve asked.

I thought about this for a while; it was a question I had asked myself not more than ten minutes before when I had been hovering over the apneic infant back in the treatment room. "It's up to you. You signed a 'do not resuscitate' order when he was in the hospital. I don't think it makes much sense to try to resuscitate him now."

"Trying to resuscitate him would probably hurt him, wouldn't it?" Nancy asked, and I nodded. "We both decided that, whatever happened, we didn't want Scotty to have to suffer."

"That's true," I responded. "But you have to do whatever you feel comfortable doing. Remember, you're going to be living with these memories for the rest of your lives. If you think you'll feel uneasy not trying to resuscitate him, if you think you'll have lingering doubt in the back of your mind in the future, then certainly you should try it. Does that make sense?"

They both nodded their heads.

"Where were we?" I asked.

"We were in the emergency room," Steve reminded me.

"Right," I continued. "The ER doctor will declare Scotty dead, and then he'll be taken down to the hospital's morgue. At that point you'll have to call a funeral home and make arrangements for the burial."

I just couldn't go on after that. The Thompsons, Steve holding his son in his arms, had both started crying. I started crying as well. We decided to end the visit at that point. After they had dried their tears and had dressed Scotty in his little coat, they headed out of my office.

THAT VISIT OCCURRED ten days ago, just before the start of this terrible week. I walked through the door of the funeral home that day feeling sadder than I had in a long time. I couldn't remember any good I'd done for anybody, the children I was caring for or their families: my patients all seemed to be steadily growing sicker, and some, like Scotty and the baby with Jarcho-Levin syndrome, had died. I realized that death was about the best I could hope for in some of these children, infants so mal-formed, so severely defective that they had virtually no chance of leading any sort of normal life. And some of the parents with whom I had dealt, parents like that couple whose newborn had Down syndrome, thoroughly resented my meddling. Yes, as I entered the funeral home that Saturday morning, I definitely felt it was time for a new career: perhaps general pediatrics, perhaps a career outside of medicine altogether.

The funeral home was packed. More than a hundred people, family and friends, had turned out to bid farewell to this tiny baby who had experienced so little of what life had to offer. Upon walking into the foyer, I immediately saw the Thomp-sons; they looked about how I expected them to look: both dressed in black, both with tears running down their cheeks. Seeing them like that caused my own problems to disappear from my mind.

Breaking away from the small group that was surround-ing her, Nancy approached me and gave me a hug. "I'm so glad you could be here, Bob," she said. Surprised and a little embar-rassed by her show of emotion, I hugged her back and heard her say, "It means a lot to us."

As she released her hold on me, I saw Steve approach and

offer his hand. Shaking it, I said, "I'm so sorry this all had to happen."

Our contact lasted only a few seconds; the Thompsons were pulled away by the director of the funeral home. It was time to start the service.

Entering the chapel, I found one of the few remaining empty seats. A small white casket, looking more like a cradle or a basinette, sat on a table at the front of the room. Steve walked to a podium that had been set to the side of the table and began to talk.

"Scotty was only with us for a short time," he began. "Just five weeks. But those five weeks have meant more to Nancy and me than any other time during our lives. For one month, we were a family; Scotty did that. He brought Nancy and me together. He brought all of us together."

Tears were spilling out of my eyes, and I felt a lump settle in my throat as I listened. Steve talked about the things that had set Scotty apart and had made him special: his bright red hair, hair so bright, Steve explained, that people could spot it a hundred yards away; the way the baby had begun to cry in recent weeks, at times when he was hungry or uncomfortable, and the way he cooed after his needs were met, sounds and reactions that indicated unequivocally to Steve and Nancy that the boy could and did respond to their interactions with him. He talked about all the good things that had come from Scotty's presence in their lives; how the extended family had unified and solidified in support of the couple, a phenomenon that no one ever thought would be possible; and how Scotty's condition had allowed them to meet a whole group of new people, how it had introduced them to, among many others, a physician who had cared for them and for their son, and had patiently helped them through what had been the most difficult period of their lives. "We owe a debt of gratitude to these people," Steve said, "a debt we'll never possibly be able to repay."

Sitting in my chair, crying freely now, listening to these words, I suddenly felt a great weight fly off me. Things began to come back into focus. I realized that through all the gloom and darkness, I really had done some good. Even though I had not healed Scotty or offered anything tangible that would improve his underlying problem or delay its inevitable outcome, I had done something important for the boy's parents. Apparently, by just being available to them, by listening to their concerns and answering their questions, I had helped them. Steve's words, uttered sadly near the end of the eulogy for his son, had renewed my spirit, giving me all the motivation I needed to begin another week and go on.

LOOKING BACK, I realize that Scotty's funeral was a turning point for me. That day I really came to understand that when caring for a child with a serious genetic disorder like trisomy 13, my patient is not necessarily only the child with the disease; the parents are also my patients, as are the child's siblings, grandparents, and extended family. And often, even though it's frustrating because there's nothing I can do for the Scottys of the world, satisfaction comes from taking care of the rest of these patients.

The day of Scotty's funeral, I also realized how clinical genetics was often a two-way street: even though I couldn't cure him, or prolong his life, or alleviate his pain, I was able to do some good for Scotty's family, to help them through the tragedy that was his death. But at the same time I came to appreciate that the parents had done some good for me. Caring for people like the Thompsons is an unbelievably satisfying experience. I feel fortunate and privileged to have had a job that, through the years, has given me the opportunity to interact in this way with so many families. These interactions have changed me, have altered my approach to my patients and their families. I hope these changes have been for the better.

CHAPTER 5

Andrew's Parents

I T'S NATURAL TO think that my years as a medical geneticist have had a major effect on how I view life. Caring for people with disabilities, witnessing firsthand the countless number of errors that can occur during embryogenesis, errors that lead to unspeakably bad outcomes, has made me more appreciative of how amazing it is when everything works out the way it's supposed to. My experience has caused me to come to value life more than I did when I was a resident. This was first driven home to me soon after Beth and I moved into the house in which we currently live.

IT WAS THE FIRST Memorial Day since we'd moved into that new house and the Gilmans, our across-the-street neighbors, invited us over for a barbecue. Since moving in two months before, we and the Gilmans had become fast friends. Our families had a lot in common. Len, a professor of biology at New York University, and I had both chosen careers in academics. His wife, Lynn, and my wife, Beth, were both teachers who had decided to put off going back to work until our kids started elementary school. And probably most significant of all, our oldest children, both three-year-old girls, had been born only weeks apart and, since our move from the Bronx, had become nearly inseparable. Late that afternoon, as we sat in deck chairs sipping beer while waiting for the charcoals in the grill to heat up, I remarked to Len on these astounding coincidences. He stopped me when I got to the part about Dori and Emily being our oldest children. "You know, Bob, Lynn and I had a child before Emily was born."

"Sure," I replied quickly, a little tipsy from the beer. "And you keep him locked up in the attic, right?"

"No," he answered almost matter-of-factly. "Andrew passed away when he was two months old."

Suddenly, I wasn't feeling all that tipsy anymore. "Oh, I'm sorry," I said, as thoughts of sudden infant death syndrome and overwhelming bacterial sepsis, the kinds of conditions that kill healthy two-month-old infants, flashed through my brain. "I had no idea. What happened?"

"We're still not exactly sure," he replied after a few seconds of hesitation. "Andrew was born ten weeks prematurely. Lynn developed hypertension. At first, her obstetricians tried to treat her with medication and bed rest, but the blood pressure wouldn't come down. Finally, they decided it would be best for everybody to deliver the baby by cesarean section. He weighed two pounds, ten ounces at birth."

"A giant," I thought, knowing from experience that in the neonatal intensive care unit, a baby of that size rarely has any serious problems.

Len continued: "At first, he had some trouble breathing, so they put him on a respirator. But he got better pretty quickly and by the time he was a week old, he was off the machine. After that, he just needed a little extra oxygen for a while.

"Those next few weeks were the best for us. Lynn and I spent as much time with Andrew as we could. Lynn would be there all day, and I'd come and join her after work. He was still too small to be able to eat on his own, he couldn't suck yet, but Lynn learned how to use the feeding tube and tried to give him all his meals. In the evening, we'd take turns holding him. By the time he was a month old, the doctors had weaned him off the extra oxygen; they told us he'd be able to come home as soon as he gained enough weight. But then he developed these episodes where he forgot to breathe."

"Apnea spells," I answered. (Apnea, literally "not breathing," is a cause of morbidity in very premature infants.)

"Right, apnea spells," Len continued. "They treated him with caffeine, but it didn't seem to do any good." (Caffeine, a methylxanthine, stimulates movement of the diaphragm in premature babies, thereby treating periodic breathing, a cause of apnea spells.) "The spells kept getting worse, and then early one morning, we got a call from the hospital that he'd taken a turn for the worst. By the time we got there, he was already gone."

Silently, I took a pull on my beer. I realized from my own experience that the story of the Gilman baby's death was very unusual. Although very premature infants, those born after only 25 or 26 weeks of gestation, often die of complications in the neonatal period, 30-weekers, as this baby had been, nearly always survive. I wondered what had gone wrong, whether Andrew's death might have been due to poor medical management. Had the doctors who'd cared for him screwed up? Had they overlooked some subtle symptom or sign, some abnormal lab result that, had it been detected, might have spared this infant's life, thereby preventing the suffering Len and Lynn had had to endure, torment that was clearly visible in the lines of my friend's face? I knew such errors occurred; since starting my internship, I'd spent enough time around intensive care nurseries to know that oversights and mistakes happen all the time. "It must have been terrible," I finally said. "There can't be anything worse than losing a child."

"You can't even imagine, Bob," Len said. "It was a nightmare. We wanted that little boy so much! The first few weeks after we buried him, I walked around in a fog. I couldn't think, I couldn't eat, I couldn't sleep. Even now when I think about it . . ." He stopped there; he just couldn't go on. I could see that his eyes had become moist.

LATER THAT NIGHT, after all the hamburgers and hot dogs had been eaten, after we'd walked back across the street to our house and put Dori and her infant sister, Davida, to bed, I asked Beth if she knew about Andrew. "Sure, I know all about him," she replied. "Lynn talks about him all the time. She's never gotten over his death."

"It's such a strange story," I said. "Babies that size nearly always survive. I wonder if someone screwed up."

"If someone screwed up, it was probably one of your old buddies," Beth replied. "Do you know where Andrew was born?"

Without waiting for my response, she continued: "University Hospital; he was born in January 1981. He died there two months later."

"My junior residency year," I said, not having to even think about it. "I worked in that NICU that year. Jesus, I might have even taken care of him."

I sat quietly for a few moments, thinking. I was really disturbed by the story; it didn't take me long to figure out why.

In March 1981, although scheduled to work in the pediatric emergency room during the day, I was assigned to take night call in the neonatal intensive care unit at University Hospital. Having already spent four months in that NICU during the course of my residency, I'd come to really detest the place. The unit featured nearly hourly medical crises, interspersed with frequent nerve-racking emergency trips to the hospital's delivery room to attend the birth of a baby believed by the obstetric staff to have the potential to enter this world with some critical illness, endless admissions of these critically ill infants to the NICU, and worst of all, the not-infrequent death of babies, all occurring in a background of never-ending, mind-numbing paperwork and follow-up tasks, known to us not so affectionately as "scut." Being on call alone at night in that NICU made me queasy, tense, insecure, and hostile.

I REMEMBER BEING particularly angry that night. It was my birthday. Nobody should have to be on call on his or her birthday! And it had been a difficult shift. By 3:00 A.M., I'd had five calls to the delivery room. Although three of them had turned out to be false alarms, with the babies coming out healthy and crying, and requiring no special assistance in transforming themselves from fetuses to newborns, the deliveries of the other two had been the stuff that makes house officers working in the NICU old before their time.

At around 2:00 A.M., I'd single-handedly resuscitated a 27-week preemie who had needed a great deal of help in making the transition to extrauterine life. I'd intubated him in the delivery room (that is, placed a tube through his mouth, past his vocal cords, and down into his trachea) and, with one of the delivery room nurses pumping oxygen into his lungs using an Ambu bag (a rubber bag attached to an oxygen supply that has a mask at one end), I'd inserted a plastic tube into one of the arteries in his umbilical cord and shot in a whole series of medications designed to keep his heart beating. I'd only just gotten that baby stabilized and settled on one of the warming tables in the NICU when I'd been summoned to the delivery room again. This time it was to attend the delivery of a full-term infant who'd passed meconium, the baby's first bowel movement, when his mother had been in labor. In the seconds after birth, this infant had sucked the green, viscous meconium deep into his lungs, making them virtually unusable for the exchange of oxygen and carbon dioxide.

These two critically ill newborns managed to hold my attention through the remainder of that night. I hadn't had time to take care of the scut work that had been signed out to me by the day crew, nor had I had a chance to even look at the two-month-old with worsening apnea and bradycardia (slowing of the heart rate) who, according to his nurse, wasn't looking quite right. And what with adjusting the ventilator settings so that the new preemie got enough oxygen into his bloodstream and holding repeated telephone discussions with the attending neonatologist who was on call that night about when to start Priscoline (tolazoline hydrochloride), a drug that decreases pulmonary resistance, on the newborn with meconium aspiration who'd developed a serious but not unexpected complication called persistence of the fetal circulation, I'd become even more frazzled and more hostile than usual. In retrospect, I'm ashamed to say that during that night I wasn't thinking of any of my charges as human; rather, they were nothing more to me than inanimate objects that had been placed in the NICU simply to torture me.

So I wasn't exactly in the best of moods when, at nearly 5:00 A.M., the nurse caring for the two-month-old with apnea and bradycardia shouted that her patient's heart had stopped beating. Dropping what I was doing, I rushed over and began working on the infant. While the nurse performed external chest compressions, I intubated him and, using an Ambu bag, began pushing oxygen directly into his lungs; we gave round after round of resuscitation medication through his intravenous line, but we simply never got him back. And when we finally decided to call it and declare him dead at around 6:00 A.M., after we'd worked on him for an entire hour without managing to get his heart to beat on its own even once, the first thought that ran through my mind was "Well, that's one less sign-out I have to do." After all, this event wasn't exactly exceptional. The child was a preemie, and preemies sometimes don't survive. True, this one was bigger and more mature than most who die, but everyone knew these children often didn't make it.

After we'd stopped working on him, I called the attending neonatologist again and told her what had happened. Clearly pissed off at me, she said she'd be in by seven and asked that the nurse call the parents and ask them to get to the hospital as soon as possible. Since the newly born preemie and the baby who had aspirated meconium were now finally stable, I spent the next hour writing admission notes and filling out a death certificate on the two-month-old. When the day crew arrived to begin their shift at a little after seven, I apologized for having failed to get their scut work done, signed out to them, and left to begin my day assignment in the emergency room. I never saw or spoke with the dead baby's parents. And on that morning, as far as I was concerned, that was perfectly fine with me.

LOOKING BACK ON it now, focusing on how I felt about all those critically ill infants whose well-being had been placed in my hands and on how I reacted to Andrew Gilman's death, I'm both amazed and ashamed at how little those lives meant to me. The fact is that when I'd been overworked and abused in that and in other intensive care units, death had seemed to be a natural, expected, even welcome part of the job. As a resident, I functioned as a technician working shifts, an automaton using machines and medications to get the patients who were assigned to me through until the next shift appeared to take charge. In those days, I had no patience for the non-technical roles that physicians were supposed to play, little understanding of just how the death of this baby might affect his parents and loved ones, and nearly no conception of how long the pain might last for these people who, after all, were so much like me and my family.

As the years have passed and the nightmare time that was my residency recedes further into my memory, I've developed a better understanding of these aspects of medicine that during my training were unimportant mysteries to me. But my progress hasn't made me feel all that comfortable. Rather, the realization of how far I've come since working in that NICU has humbled me. After all, if I had so little concept of the significance of the lives of my patients back then, what will I think about the way I practice medicine in the future? What will I know then, learned through the experience of more years of caring for children and their families that I can't even conceive of at the present? Unable to answer any of these questions, all I can do is try my best, understanding that, as judged from the perspective of the future, my best today is almost certain to fall short of the mark.

A few days after our Memorial Day barbecue, I told Len that I'd been the resident on call the night Andrew had died. He didn't say a word in response, only nodded his head and quickly changed the topic. Nearly a quarter of a century has passed since that day, and neither he nor I have ever mentioned the events surrounding Andrew's death again. For Len, it must be the pain that prevents him from talking about it. For me, it's simply the embarrassment I feel whenever I think of the way I acted during that long night on call.

ALTHOUGH THE REALIZATION that I had been on call the night Andrew Gilman died was an important event in my evolution as a physician, it was only one of many. Probably the most significant event occurred about five years after that Memorial Day barbecue, at the same University Hospital. At that time, at about 36 weeks of gestation, Beth delivered a stillborn baby. Although the pregnancy had gone extremely well, with no complications whatsoever, two days before she delivered, Beth noticed that the baby had just stopped moving. That was all; one moment she was kicking and punching, the next there was nothing. We went to the labor and delivery floor, where a sonogram revealed that for no rhyme or reason, with no plausible explanation that anyone could offer, our baby's heart had stopped beating; the fetus had simply died in the womb. Beth delivered her two days later, we named her Orly Shira, had a funeral, and tried to go on with our lives.

And we've succeeded. But every so often, especially in early spring when the cherry tree we planted in our backyard in her memory comes into full bloom, we take out the envelope bearing the few keepsakes of her existence (a few photos, the hat that was put on her head, her death certificate) and we think about what she might be like today. Unfortunately, we'll never know.

My experience with families like the Gilmans, as well as the events that have occurred in my own life, have shown me that in practicing medicine (and clinical genetics in particular), providing for the emotional needs of the family both at the time of the initial encounter and then on an ongoing basis, can be as important (if not more important) than the provision of physical care. This may be the biggest epiphany I've experienced during the years I've been in practice. As occurred in the case of the Thompsons (but didn't occur in the case of the Gilmans), by attending to families' emotional needs, doctors can provide crucial services—services that go above and beyond those that are taught in medical school and in residency training.

CHAPTER 6

September 11, 3:00 P.M.

I HAD BEEN SITTING at my desk for only a few minutes when the phone rang. Although it was the first time I'd heard a phone ring in a long time, I was so caught up in my own thoughts that I ignored the sound. But then Billie, my secretary, knocked on the door. "The clinic's on the phone," she said. "Your three o'clock patient's here."

"A patient showed up?" I replied. "Didn't they cancel everyone?"

"The phones weren't working," she said. "They didn't expect anyone to show up, but here she is."

I checked the schedule that was sitting atop the pile of charts on my desk. "Brandy Guzman," I read. "A nine-month-old with Down syndrome coming for routine follow-up. She doesn't even need to be seen! What the hell is she doing coming in on a day like this?"

"Do you want them to reschedule?" Billie asked.

"No," I said after some slight hesitation. "Something must

be going on with the mom. I'll see her." And then I tried to gather the energy needed to rise out of my chair and walk to the clinic building.

I HAD NO ENERGY. It had been one of the worst days in the history of the world. The morning had started out like every other morning that September. It had been the first day of the second week of my obligatory month of attending rounds on the Children's Hospital's infants' floor. The ward had been quiet for the past week, and that morning only 16 of the 26 beds were occupied. To help fill up the time, I'd prepared a talk for the residents on common chromosomal disorders for attending rounds that morning, and at a little before 8:00 A.M., I'd stopped by my office to pick up some slides. Then I'd headed to Morning Report, the daily conference run by the chief residents at which all the patients who had been admitted the day before were discussed.

Morning Report had been calm, almost boring; only three children had come onto the entire pediatric service the night before, and all had had respiratory distress resulting from exacerbation of their asthma. Near the end of the conference, I remember thinking how easy the day was going to be: a few minutes discussing our patients (none of whom were particularly sick); a few minutes talking about Down syndrome, trisomy 13 and 18, and a few other chromosomal disorders; and then I'd be free to go about my own business, getting ready for the patients I was scheduled to see that afternoon in clinic. But then Morning Report ended and I walked out of the conference room to find that the world had changed forever.

In the hall leading to the staircase, I was stopped by Amanda Sterman, one of the interns on our team. "Dr. Marion, did you hear what happened?" she asked. "Two jets flew into the World Trade Center."

"What?" I asked, not fully processing the information she was giving me. "How did that happen? Was it an accident?"

"No. They're saying it was a terrorist attack. And there are other attacks going on. The Pentagon's been hit; the Supreme Court Building is under attack. And there are other planes that can't be accounted for."

In silence, Amanda and I took the staircase down to the ward. I found the entire staff—residents, interns, medical students, nurses, clerks, and orderlies—huddled around the TV in the nurses' lounge, watching images on the screen that just didn't make sense. The twin towers of the World Trade Center, enormous buildings located barely ten miles from where I stood, structures that on a clear day were visible from the windows of the south-facing patient rooms, had been transformed into funeral pyres, burning out of control. In the room, except for the sound of the reporters' voices, there was total silence; every person bore a look of shock on his or her face.

I joined this scene, immediately becoming absorbed by the images. Within a minute of my arrival, as my brain was only just beginning to interpret the significance of those images, one of our chief residents hurried onto the floor. He told us that the hospital's administration had ordered that the emergency action plan be initiated. Because of our proximity to the World Trade Center, it was expected that sometime during the afternoon a flood of injured people would spill over from the hospitals in Manhattan into our emergency department. To prepare for this eventuality, we were to do two things. First, in an attempt to free up as many beds as possible, we were to release all inpatients who could safely be discharged to home. Second, we were all to stand by and await further instructions.

Our team, already frustrated by our inability to do anything to help, was only too happy to follow these orders. The senior resident, charge nurse, and I walked the floor, making decisions about who could go home and who should stay. In each room, every TV was tuned to the same station, now the only one that the hospital's televisions seemed to be able to receive, spilling out the same images. Mothers and fathers, holding their babies, watched the twin towers burn. Many of them cried.

In each room, we tried to calm them, to offer some comfort and support, but what could we say? The mother of a two-year-old boy who'd been admitted early that morning with asthma was the most upset. She worked in an office on the 38th floor of one of the towers and was friends with more than a dozen people who should have been in the building that morning; had her child not been in the hospital, she, too, would have been there. Since the first bulletin had been broadcast, she'd been trying to call her office, but the phones weren't working; when she called, all she heard was a rapid busy signal. As time passed, she was becoming more frantic, and nothing we could do or say could calm her. As her wailing and agitation increased, her son's respiratory distress worsened. Ultimately, we gave her 10 milligrams of Valium (diazepam); it was the only way to get her to calm down.

By discharging all who were stable or near stable, we were able to reduce our census from 16 to 6. We'd complied with the chief resident's first order. To fulfill the second, our staff sat in that small nurses' lounge and waited for the stream of patients to be transported in.

We waited . . . and waited . . . and waited.

It was terrible. None of us had lived through anything like this. We'd never served as care providers in a time of crisis, and we didn't know what to expect. We realized that there weren't likely to be many children in the World Trade Center. Would young casualties from the surrounding areas, children from local schools and day care centers, be brought to us? Would we be called on to care for injured adults? Or worse, would we be left with nothing to do, no patients either young or old, because no one had survived?

We tried not to think of this final, horrible scenario. We just waited, passing the time watching the events play out on TV. We watched the buildings burn, we watched the towers fall, we watched the crowds run, we tried to support one another.

Fortunately, none of us had friends or relatives who were in lower Manhattan that morning. But all had loved ones somewhere in the area, and we each attempted to call them, to be comforted by hearing their voices. I tried to reach my wife, who was at work at a high school in Westchester County, about 25 miles north of the Trade Center; I tried to call my daughters, who were at colleges in upstate New York; I tried to call my father, who was across the river in New Jersey. In no case was I successful: the telephone system had been devastated, another casualty of the disaster.

At about 2:00 P.M., burned out from the now five hours of waiting, I walked down to the pediatric emergency room to see what was happening. The scene I found there was perhaps the second most upsetting sight I'd seen that day. As part of the emergency action plan, all members of the ER staff had been called in. Despite the monumental traffic problems and security issues, most had managed to make it to the hospital. But after arriving, they had little to do. Not a single patient had been transported from what was now being called Ground Zero; no one had come from Manhattan for emergency care of any kind; in fact, the usual emergencies that are a constant part of life in our hospital had stopped arriving. So the staff had set up chairs in the trauma area, and that's where I found them, the entire staff, sitting and watching TV. No one was working. The place was dead.

That's when I realized for sure that there weren't going to be any survivors of this terrible attack. Rather than going back to the ward to take up my place in front of the TV, rather than staying at my post, awaiting patients who were never going to arrive, I went back to my office, closed the door, sat at my desk, buried my head in my hands, and began to sob. I'd been at my desk for barely ten minutes when the telephone rang, telling me that Brandy Guzman had arrived for her three o'clock follow-up appointment.

WALKING TO THE CLINIC, I tried to pull myself together so that I could focus on the task at hand. Brandy was the first child born to her mother, Jessica Guzman. I'd been called to see the baby immediately after birth because the staff had been concerned that she had Down syndrome. And they'd been correct: Brandy had all the external features of trisomy 21. When I met with Jessica, who was 24 at the time, she'd become extremely upset, so upset that I'd had to call the maternity unit's social worker to help me. Together, we'd managed to calm the new mother. But right from that beginning, I'd had real concerns about this woman's ability to deal with the crisis she was about to experience.

Brandy had turned out to be healthy. After a workup had revealed that she had no internal malformations, such as congenital heart disease or duodenal atresia (a malformation of the small intestine), and since she'd had no problem feeding, she'd left the hospital on the third day of life. When our genetic counselor and I met with Jessica and her own mother, Myra, with whom she and the baby lived, to show them the infant's chromosome analysis a few days later, the young woman again became extremely upset, breaking down in tears, crying and wailing uncontrollably. We spent more than two hours speaking with her, again eventually succeeding in calming her. Myra had been very helpful during that session; I remember feeling relieved that someone so mature and responsible would be involved with this baby's care.

Over the next few months, I saw Brandy in the clinic virtually every other week. During that time I had no concerns about the child's health; an infant who fed and grew well and had no significant illnesses, Brandy needed very little support from us. No, those visits weren't for Brandy; they were for Jessica. I was concerned about how the mother was coping with her daughter's condition. And it had been rough sledding for a long time.

But as the months passed, Jessica clearly improved. She came to see that Brandy was a beautiful baby, and much like other infants in most ways. We referred the baby to a New York State certified early intervention program, and mother and child had attended faithfully. The mother's improvement was a relief to me: I came to see that both she and her daughter were going to make it through this. And on my way to the clinic that afternoon, looking at the chart, I noted that the last time I'd seen Brandy or heard from Jessica or her mother was a full three months before, when they'd come for the child's six-month visit.

Brandy and Jessica were the only people sitting in the waiting area. Brandy was sleeping peacefully in her stroller; Jessica was crying quietly. Walking up to them, I put my arm on Jessica's shoulder and asked what was wrong.

"My mother . . ." was all she was able to get out, and my heart sank. I hadn't remembered until then that Myra worked at the World Trade Center.

"You haven't heard from her?"

She shook her head.

"Why did you leave home? What if she tries to call you—"

She cut me off by pointing to her cell phone.

With my arm around her, I virtually carried Jessica from the waiting area into one of the treatment rooms. One of the clerks pushed the baby's stroller behind us. "What's her phone number?" I asked, and Jessica, still not able to speak, wrote it on a piece of paper on the desk in front of us, her hands shaking as she scribbled the numbers. Although I was successful in getting a dial tone, when I punched in the number of Myra's office, all I heard was that rapid busy signal. "I'm not getting through," I said. Jessica's crying crescendoed. I knew I had to do something. But what?

I called everyone I could think of calling. I called hospital security; although the person who answered the phone was sympathetic, he told me there was nothing he could do. I called 911; the first two times I got nothing, but the third time I managed to reach an operator. She told me that, although she also could do little, she'd take Myra's name and our phone number and would call if anything turned up. Using the phone book, I tried calling the emergency rooms of the hospitals closest to the World Trade Center: Beekman Downtown, St. Luke's–Roosevelt, and on and on. I managed to get through to none of them. As time passed—15 minutes, then 20, then 30—my frustration level rose. But amazingly, Jessica's crying seemed to come under control during this time.

"Do you know why I came to this visit today, Dr. Marion?" she asked as I was checking the phone book for yet another number to try.

"Brandy had an appointment?" I responded.

"Well, that was part of it," she answered. "But it was because I knew you'd be here for me. You helped me so much when Brandy was first born. I knew you would help me now. . . ." And she started crying again.

Putting down the phone, I wrapped my arms around her, this young woman who could have been my own daughter, and began softly crying myself.

I don't know how long we sat like that, but the silence was broken by the sound of a phone ringing. It was Jessica's cell phone. She picked it up and heard the voice of her mother.

Myra had made it out of the building. With a crowd of other people, she'd run north to safety. Although she was safe, she was stuck in midtown Manhattan with no way of getting home and no method of contacting anyone. She'd been trying all day to reach Jessica, to let her know that she was all right, but her cell phone just wouldn't work. Finally, after hours of trying, she'd managed to get through.

The visit ended with Brandy still sleeping in her stroller. Jessica, her face washed, her crying finished, thanked me and headed home. I sat in the silent treatment room by myself for a good 15 minutes, reflecting on what had happened that day. And then I got out of my chair and headed for the parking lot.

CHAPTER 7

Relics

W E MEDICAL GENETICISTS play many roles in the lives of our patients. We're the bearers of news, both good and bad, about the health and well-being of children and potential future children. We're a source of information that can help in decision making about couples' reproductive future and serve as a sounding board once those decisions have been made. We offer support during crises and with time can become a trusted member of our patients' extended families. And as in cases like that of Melissa Moore, we can use our knowledge to provide answers to questions and solve problems. This was definitely the case when the Kennedys came to see me.

"YOU TWO ARE MEETING us for the first time. You don't know us at all, but there's something about us you have to understand," Mr. Kennedy told me and Carol Stern, one of the genetic counselors with whom I work. "My wife and I, we believe strongly that all life is sacred and that abortion is wrong. But after having to stand by and watch our daughter, our only child, deteriorate and die the way she did, with us not being able to do anything to help her, we just could never go through anything like that again. So unless there's some way you can guarantee that this baby won't be affected, unless you can tell us for sure that everything will be all right, we're going to have to go ahead and do what we were originally planning to do."

It was the first time the Kennedys had come to our office, and Carol and I were engrossed by their story. The couple had been referred by an obstetrician; Elaine Kennedy, a 28-year-old woman, was then in the tenth week of her second pregnancy, a pregnancy that had come as a surprise to both her and her husband. Following the death of their first child, Sarah, the Kennedys had vowed never to risk having another baby.

The story the Kennedys told us that day was not unusual for the disease that had affected Sarah. The child, who'd been born after a completely normal, uncomplicated pregnancy, had been delivered in a hospital in North Carolina, where the family had been living. A beautiful baby who seemed perfect in every way, Sarah had left the hospital on the second day of life, having been declared healthy by the family's pediatrician.

But this perfect beginning quickly gave way to a period of confusion and complications. Problems began during Sarah's third week of life. Her parents noticed that the infant was having trouble feeding: where initially she'd been able to gobble down three or four ounces of formula in just a few minutes, it now was taking longer for her to finish her bottle. During her one-month checkup, the Kennedys brought this to the attention of their pediatrician, who noted a lack of weight gain in

Sarah and also became concerned. On examining the baby, the doctor saw that the infant's muscle tone was extremely low. Calling Sarah a "floppy baby," he referred the child for evaluation to Dr. Fred Wilmot, a well-known pediatric neurologist at the Duke University Medical Center in Durham.

In the two weeks between the visit to the pediatrician and the appointment with the neurologist, Sarah became weaker with each passing day. Although she now smiled when she saw her parents, she could no longer lift her head off the mattress of her crib. And feeding her became a real chore: the Kennedys spent nearly all their time trying to get enough calories into their daughter to sustain her. By the time they were sitting in the neurologist's waiting room in Durham, they had both come to realize that something was seriously wrong with their daughter.

Dr. Wilmot knew immediately what that something was. Upon hearing the story and observing the girl's activity, her obvious attentiveness to her parents' voices but her nearly total lack of any voluntary muscle movement, he told the couple he was concerned that Sarah had a condition called spinal muscular atrophy. A few days later that diagnosis was confirmed when muscle tissue obtained during a biopsy of Sarah's thigh showed the characteristic changes seen in this disease.

PUT SIMPLY, a diagnosis of the infantile form of spinal muscular atrophy (SMA) is a death sentence. A relatively rare disease in which the nerves that control all the voluntary muscles of the body slowly and mysteriously disappear, it is a degenerative condition, the childhood equivalent of the better-known, but also poorly understood, amyotrophic lateral sclerosis

(ALS), more commonly known as Lou Gehrig's disease after the New York Yankees first baseman who died of the condition. As the nerves vanish during the first months of life, the child with SMA becomes progressively weaker. After initial problems with feeding, the infant ceases to be able to move the arms or legs; breathing becomes progressively more difficult, the child becoming more and more hungry for air until finally, by about the first birthday, the child dies, usually as a result of aspiration pneumonia. During the course of the disease, the infant's intelligence remains intact; trapped inside an increasingly useless body, he or she seems totally aware of what is happening.

Sarah Kennedy lived such a nightmarish existence. On the day the diagnosis was confirmed, after they'd sat in Dr. Wilmot's office and heard the terrible news, her parents took their daughter home and tried to go on as if nothing had happened. But the Kennedys couldn't keep the reality away for long. By four months, Sarah, now completely unable to suck or swallow, was being fed formula through a nasogastric tube, a piece of plastic inserted through her nose that passed into her esophagus and down into her stomach. By six months, she was completely paralyzed, with only her eyes—which remained alert and focused and filled with normal baby intelligence—letting on that she was still alive. During her eighth month, a bout of pneumonia nearly caused her death. It was during the hospitalization that followed, an ordeal that lasted three weeks, that the Kennedys made the most difficult decision any parent can ever make: they signed a "do not resuscitate" order, agreeing with the doctors who were treating Sarah that no heroic efforts should be made to keep their daughter alive. Mercifully, Sarah died peacefully at home, in her sleep, on the day of her ten-month birthday.

Although the Kennedys were devastated by Sarah's illness and by her death, the baby's funeral was not the end of their nightmare. During the session when he told them of Sarah's diagnosis, Dr. Wilmot informed the Kennedys that because of the way SMA is inherited, each subsequent child born to the couple had a one-in-four chance of also being affected. An autosomal recessively inherited condition, SMA results from the presence of two copies of a nonfunctioning gene in the affected child. The parents of such children, who are carriers, each bear one copy of the nonfunctioning gene and another copy of the gene that functions normally; the single functioning gene is enough to prevent them from developing symptoms. When a carrier father produces sperm or a carrier mother makes eggs, each has a one-in-two chance of including the nonfunctioning gene. Thus, when the sperm and egg combine, there is one chance out of four that the child will receive both nonfunctioning genes, a situation that would result in an affected child.

During that session, Dr. Wilmot gave the Kennedys one more piece of devastating news: because the actual gene responsible for SMA had not yet been localized to a specific chromosome within the enormous human genome, prenatal detection of the condition was not possible; there was no way of predicting whether the couple's next child would be affected with the disease until after that child was born and either developed symptoms as Sarah had, or having sailed through the first few months of life unscathed, could be declared free of the condition. Then and only then, the neurologist told them, would the Kennedys be able to breathe comfortably.

So, gradually, once the shock of Sarah's diagnosis wore off, once they managed to work through the unbearable news that their beautiful daughter would most probably not survive her first year of life, the Kennedys began to discuss the future. By the time Sarah was seven months old, after they'd watched her suffer more with each passing day, helpless to do anything to alleviate that suffering, the couple decided that they could not live through this nightmare again. Rather than take the chance, the Kennedys decided that after Sarah's death they would remain childless.

And that's the way it had been. For more than three years, by being careful, Mrs. Kennedy had managed to avoid getting pregnant. But then, a few weeks before their meeting with us, as a result of fate, bad luck, carelessness, or a combination of all three, Mrs. Kennedy had missed her period. She informed her husband about the news only after a home pregnancy test came out positive. And thus began the current crisis in the lives of these people.

During the first part of our counseling session, the Kennedys had explained how ambivalent they felt about the pregnancy. On the one hand, Mrs. Kennedy said, in the years since Sarah's death, they'd come to view their lives as empty, missing an important component. They had applied to adoption agencies, but the waiting lists were long and they were afraid they were still years away from success; they'd placed ads in newspapers around the country, trying to reach women who were interested in giving up a child for adoption, but nothing had ever come of it. They had considered the possibility of artificial insemination using sperm from an anonymous donor, but they had rejected this option because they felt that not knowing for sure whether the donor was a carrier of the gene for SMA was still too risky.

Although it was clear that the Kennedys desperately wanted the child then developing in Mrs. Kennedy's uterus, it was also clear how much they feared that 25 percent risk of recurrence. So when the pregnancy test had turned out positive, they'd sought out an obstetrician affiliated with our hospital in hopes of obtaining a first-trimester abortion. Upon hearing the story and recognizing the couple's ambivalence, that doctor had referred the Kennedys to us, suggesting that they speak with a geneticist before consenting to perform the procedure. That's how they wound up sitting in my office that day, sharing their sad story one more time with yet another set of strangers.

AFTER MR. KENNEDY completed his impassioned statement, Carol and I remained silent for a few moments. We all needed a chance to gain control over ourselves again. Then, as Carol and I had discussed before the session had started, she began to speak: "We're happy you came to see us before doing anything, because there may be something we can do to help. Things have been changing pretty quickly in genetics. A lot has happened since Sarah passed away. Dr. Wilmot was right when he told you that the location of the gene that causes SMA wasn't known, and back then there really wasn't anything anyone could do to diagnose the condition before the symptoms actually occurred. But a couple of years ago, the gene responsible for causing SMA was mapped to a portion of chromosome 5. So although we still don't know exactly what's wrong with the gene or why a defect in it causes the disease, in some cases, rather than having to rely on clinical symptoms and the muscle biopsy for making a diagnosis, we can actually do a blood test and tell with some certainty whether a child has the disease or not."

"Are you saying that you'll be able to tell whether our baby has SMA or not?" Mrs. Kennedy asked.

"We're getting a little ahead of ourselves," Carol answered, "but the answer is 'possibly.' Each of you has two copies of chromosome 5 in every cell of your body. By doing some complicated testing on your blood called linkage analysis, it might be possible to tell which of your chromosome 5s carries the nonworking gene and which carries the working one."

"So if you know which one carries the nonworking gene, you can test the fetus and find out how many nonworking genes it has, right?" Mr. Kennedy asked. The gloom that had predominated in the room until this moment began to lift slightly. "That means you can tell if the baby will have SMA, doesn't it?"

"Basically that's right," I replied. "By doing an amniocentesis, we could get cells from the fetus and analyze them to see which copies of chromosome 5 were contributed by each of you. But there's one problem: in order to tell which of the chromosome 5s carries the nonworking gene, we need a sample of Sarah's DNA."

"A sample of Sarah's DNA?" Mrs. Kennedy asked, the optimism dying back a little. "How is that possible? How can we get a sample of DNA from a baby who's been dead for three years?"

"It might be a problem," I replied, "but in some cases in the past, we've been able to do it. Sometimes the doctors who care for a child with an inherited condition who's terminally ill will take some blood and store away the DNA so that it might be used for testing in the future. It's called DNA banking. Do you know if any of Sarah's doctors did that?"

The Kennedys looked at each other sadly. "Not that we know of," Mr. Kennedy responded.

"Maybe they did it and didn't tell us," Mrs. Kennedy added quickly, almost pleading. "Maybe you should check with Dr. Wilmot."

"We definitely will," I told them.

"And Sarah had a muscle biopsy to confirm her diagnosis," Carol said. "In some cases, we've been able to get DNA from the tissue preserved on the microscope slides. I'll call the lab that performed the test and see if we can get our hands on the slides."

"And if all that fails, there is still one other option, although it's not very nice. It's possible to exhume the body in order to get a sample of tissue," I said. When I saw the looks on the faces of the Kennedys, I quickly added, "We would only do that as a last resort, if there is no other possible way."

"I'm already in my tenth week," Mrs. Kennedy said, patting her belly, which at least externally showed no signs of her pregnant state. "Is it really reasonable to think that all this can be done in time for us to make a decision?"

"We'll do our best" was all I could tell her.

Carol remained in my office after the Kennedys had departed. "There's got to be something we can do for these people," the genetic counselor said. "They want this baby so badly. There must be some way we can get our hands on Sarah's DNA."

"I'm not optimistic," I replied. "If they weren't told anything about it, I'm pretty sure the neurologist didn't bank any DNA. What would be the purpose of banking it if the parents don't even know it's available?"

"That's true," Carol replied. "What about the biopsy slides?"

"That biopsy must have been done nearly four years ago," I answered. "I don't think labs keep slides around for that long."

"So you think we might wind up having to exhume the body?" the counselor asked.

"I'm afraid so," I said. "But that's not going to be easy. You saw their faces when I brought it up as a possibility; they looked like they'd seen a ghost. With all the emotional turmoil that goes with it and all the legal paperwork that has to get done, I'm not sure we're going to have enough time to get them an answer while they still can make a decision about abortion."

"I guess we'd better get on it," Carol said, rising and walking toward the door.

"I guess," I answered.

OVER THE NEXT few days, Carol and I tried everything we could to track down a specimen of DNA from Sarah Kennedy, but all attempts ultimately led to dead ends. For a day and a half, I played telephone tag with Dr. Wilmot. When I finally got to speak with him, he told me that, yes, he remembered Sarah Kennedy and her parents quite well, and that although he'd never heard of doing it before (and hadn't done it in this case), he thought the idea of banking DNA from patients with terminal, inherited conditions was an excellent one. "I can certainly see how such a specimen would be helpful in family planning," he told me in his southern drawl. Unfortunately, it would not be helpful in this case.

Meanwhile, Carol had her hands full with the Surgical Pathology Department at Duke University in Durham, the unit that had processed and read the muscle biopsy specimen. On the first day of her contact with Durham, a secretary told her that under no circumstances were slides in the department's files ever released to the public. When she asked to speak with the secretary's supervisor, Carol heard a click on the line; the secretary had hung up on her. Immediately calling back, Carol spoke with another secretary who did put her through to the office's administrator. But the news from that administrator was no more helpful than what she'd heard from the first secretary. What Carol had been told by the first secretary was incorrect: in certain situations, such as when a second opinion was requested, specimen slides most definitely were released. But Carol's brightened mood was darkened again, however, by the next bit of news from the administrator: slides from muscle biopsies, she was told, were retained by the archives for only three years. After that time they were promptly disposed of. Since the biopsy on the Kennedy baby had been performed four years before, the administrator was almost certain that the slides would not be found.

Carol, becoming desperate, tried as best as she could to draw the administrator in, attempting to marshal her assistance in the search for those biopsy slides. The genetic counselor recounted the sad saga of the Kennedy family, explaining how important getting our hands on those slides could be. The administrator, moved by the story but still pessimistic, told Carol that although she was almost sure the search would prove fruitless, she would personally spend some time that afternoon trying to locate the slides. She took our number and told Carol that she'd call her back the next day with the information.

She did look and she did call us back, but the news was not good. As she'd expected, the microscope slides were nowhere to be found. Sadly, Carol entered my office to tell me the news. "Where do we go from here?" she asked.

"Our only option is to exhume the body," I answered. "We'd better call the Kennedys in to bring them up-to-date on what's going on."

THE KENNEDYS WERE back in our office the next day. Glumly, Carol and I recounted what had transpired over the previous days. The couple, who had entered my office full of hope, became more anxious with each word. "Unfortunately, it looks like exhumation is our only option," I said. "Getting a body exhumed isn't easy, but with your help we'll try to do it as painlessly as possible for everyone involved."

"There's absolutely no other way?" Mrs. Kennedy asked. "Nothing else we can try?"

"Nothing I can think of," I replied. Having stopped by the office of the hospital's attorney that morning and picked up the necessary forms, I began to fill them out.

"We've been thinking about this constantly since we left

here the other day," Mr. Kennedy said in the direction of Carol. "After she died, we put a bunch of Sarah's things in a box. We brought it with us when we moved from North Carolina, and we keep it in a closet in our spare bedroom. Sometimes, like on her birthday or when we really miss her, we take the stuff out and look through it. We've got pictures, clothes, her hairbrush, her baby blanket, a rattle, things like that. I know there's nothing we can do to bring Sarah back, but just holding these things, just having these relics around makes us feel closer to her. That's the closest we can ever get to her now. They are the things that are Sarah to us now. It's a shame we can't use any of those things to do this testing."

Carol remained silent, thinking through the words that Mr. Kennedy had just said. It hit her suddenly. "Tell me the things you have in that box again," she said, with an expression that made me look up from the paperwork.

"Photographs of Sarah," the father began, counting off each item on the fingers of his left hand, "some of the clothes she wore during the last few weeks of her life, her hairbrush—"

"Stop right there," Carol ordered. "Have you cleaned the hair out of the brush?"

"No," Mrs. Kennedy replied, shaking her head. "We couldn't. It's . . . it's the only piece of her we have left."

"Exactly," Carol said, now getting excited. "It's a piece of Sarah. And it may contain enough DNA to allow us to do the testing. Can you bring it to us right away?"

The Kennedys were back in our office an hour later, bearing a brown paper bag. Inside the bag was an infant's-size pink plastic hairbrush; packed within the bristles of the brush were strands of dirty-blond hair. After I'd drawn samples of blood from both parents, we placed the brush and the tubes of blood in a Styrofoam container and shipped it off to a lab in Birmingham, Alabama, that was doing linkage analysis using a molecular technique known as restriction fragment length polymorphisms to diagnose SMA. While the Kennedys had been home getting Sarah's brush, Carol had called the genetic counselor who worked with a molecular geneticist in that lab in Alabama, explaining the situation. Although she hadn't been optimistic, Carol said they would do their best with the hair specimen; she also promised to return the brush unharmed.

All that remained now was the wait. Although the time passed slowly for me, it was sheer agony for Carol and the Kennedys, who spoke with each other at least once a day. After two and a half weeks, the call finally came from the genetic counselor in Alabama. It was good news: not only had they been able to retrieve enough DNA from the hair trapped within the bristles of Sarah's brush, but the testing revealed that the family was informative. That is, they thought there was an excellent chance we'd be able to confirm or rule out SMA in the fetus.

And so, in her 15th week of pregnancy, rather than having an abortion, Mrs. Kennedy underwent an amniocentesis without complication. A week later, cultured cells obtained from that amnio were sent by overnight express to the lab in Alabama. And one week after that, word came back that the fetus had inherited one nonworking copy of the gene from his mother and one working gene from his father. The lab predicted that the baby, who we now knew would be a boy, would not be affected with SMA. Like his mother and father, the tests predicted that he would turn out to be a carrier.

And the prediction of the lab in Alabama turned out to be correct. Five months after the amniocentesis had been performed, Mrs. Kennedy gave birth to a perfect seven-pound, four-ounce baby boy. The baby, named Sean after his sister, came to visit Carol and me in our office three weeks after his birth. Robust and active, with a loud cry and a suck that just wouldn't quit, the infant showed no signs of the condition that had claimed his sister's life.

The Kennedys, though looking as if they could use a good night's sleep, were beside themselves with happiness. "Through all those dark days, I never thought anything this wonderful would ever happen to us," Mrs. Kennedy told us as she nursed her son.

Like so many couples who have lost a child, like Beth and I had done with our stillborn daughter, Orly, the Kennedys had saved pieces of their daughter's life, relics that, through the years, they hoped would ensure that memories of Sarah would live on. Unfortunately, in most cases these boxes and envelopes—kept in closets and drawers, in basements and spare bedrooms and studies—gather nothing but dust; with the passage of time, as lives become filled out with other children and other activities, they tend to see the light of day less and less, ultimately becoming forgotten forever. These remembrances almost never bear fruit. But in the case of Sarah Kennedy, a relic from her life bore the most delicious fruit in the world: out of the depths of despair, her hairbrush provided the key that allowed her brother to be born. Could there be a better testament to a dead child?

Postscript

I'D LIKE TO SAY that it was our brilliant deductive reasoning, our Sherlock Holmesian approach to the case that allowed Carol and me to make the breakthrough that ultimately led to our being able to offer the Kennedys a test that allowed them to continue their pregnancy. I'd like to say that, but I can't; sometimes, it's just dumb luck that allows you to realize you've found an answer. It's like finding a parking space in a crowded lot: sometimes you get lucky and you find the spot right in front of the entrance to the mall; other times, you wind up walking what seems like miles. In working with the Kennedys, we got the space in front of the entrance.

The genetic aspects of this essay are now extremely dated: in 1995, a group from Paris identified the gene for SMA.[1] Called *SMN* (for *survival motor neuron*), as predicted, the gene was located within a segment of DNA on the long arm of chromosome 5. The Parisian group also demonstrated changes in the gene in 226 of 229 patients with SMA, thus confirming that this was the responsible bit of DNA.

This breakthrough was a godsend for families like the Kennedys. Identification of the gene responsible for SMA made direct DNA analysis (in which mutations in the gene could be searched for in the individual at risk) a reality. No longer was it necessary to have a sample of DNA from an affected family member. Currently, in hopes of providing families with genetic counseling before they've had a child with this condition, a large-scale carrier screening program for SMA is being considered. These are huge accomplishments!

The Kennedys have clearly benefited from these revolutionary changes. After Sean was born, Mrs. Kennedy became pregnant two additional times. In each case, an amniocentesis demonstrated that the fetuses were not affected with SMA (one child was a carrier of the nonworking gene; the other inherited two copies of the working gene). Today, they have three healthy and happy children.

It's kind of ironic: in its early days, amniocentesis, in fact the entire field of medical genetics, was considered something of a search-and-destroy mission. Tests were performed on amniotic fluid cells; abnormalities were identified; and since no treatment was available, couples were offered little choice but to either terminate the pregnancies or continue on, knowing that they were destined to deliver a baby with serious problems. But the reality of the situation has always been much more like the story of the Kennedy family: without these genetic breakthroughs coupled with our ability to detect genetic disorders prenatally, couples with SMA and other inherited disorders would remain childless. The ability to test for the presence of SMA in Sean and his younger brother and sister allowed this family to have three children who otherwise would never have been born. This is one of the important reasons that, in spite of the sadness and angst associated with this field, we clinical geneticists continue to do what we do.

CHAPTER 8

The Baby Who Stopped Eating

"I SAVED THE MOST interesting case for last," said Molly Wilson, the resident who'd been on call the night before. It was a Saturday morning in early February and we were standing outside one of the patient rooms on the Children's Hospital's infants' unit. Molly, the rest of the ward team, and I had spent the last hour touring the ward, stopping to discuss and examine each child who was unlucky enough to be an inpatient on the unit that day. Concentrating, I was trying to take in all the facts and figures that were being tossed at me, but it seemed to be a losing battle. I was tired, the day was cold and gray, and I'd have much rather been home in bed than in the hospital. But as the ward's designated attending physician of the month, the senior doctor on the service, it was my job to make sure that these children were getting the best care possible, and so, fighting off the urge to daydream, I tried to refocus my attention on the resident's words.

"This baby's name is Jarrett Fox," Molly continued. "He's a three-month-old who was admitted last night for treatment of dehydration. According to his mother, Jarrett stopped eating four days before admission."

"Stopped eating?" I repeated, quickly coming to full attention. "What do you mean he stopped eating?"

"Just that," the resident replied. "His mother says that he was fine a week ago, happy and healthy and acting like a normal baby. Then, on Tuesday, he seemed to lose interest in nursing. His mother said he just stopped sucking. He hasn't eaten anything since then."

"That can't be right," I responded. "Three-month-olds don't just suddenly stop nursing and starve themselves until they get dehydrated."

"Well, that's what the mother told me," Molly replied. "I didn't believe it either, so I asked her to describe what happened three separate times, and each time she told me the same story. She's been trying to force-feed him since Wednesday, but hasn't had any success. Yesterday, not knowing what else to do, she brought him to her pediatrician, who found him to be about 5 percent dehydrated. He also said the kid was much floppier than he'd been the last time he'd seen him. So he sent him in for rehydration and a full evaluation."

That last part of Molly's report, the part about the increased floppiness, made my heart sink. It suggested a diagnosis I hoped this baby didn't have. "Do you have any ideas about a diagnosis?" I asked.

"The only thing I can think of is spinal muscular atrophy," Molly said.

"That's what I'm thinking, too," I replied. "I hope we're wrong. Let's go see him."

SPINAL MUSCULAR ATROPHY, the condition that caused the death of the Sarah Kennedy, is a death sentence. As was illustrated in the story of Sarah's life, initial problems with feeding, similar to the type Molly Wilson described in the case of Jarrett Fox, the infant loses the ability to move all of his or her muscles. Breathing becomes difficult, the child more and more air hungry, until he or she dies around the first birthday, usually as a result of pneumonia. And perhaps worst of all, during the course of the disease, the infant, trapped inside an increasingly useless body, seems totally aware of what is happening.

By that Saturday in February, I'd already been involved in the care of more than a dozen patients who had succumbed to this disease. As I entered Jarrett Fox's hospital room, I was hoping that this child wouldn't be another one added to this roster.

"MS. FOX," MOLLY SAID as we approached Jarrett's crib, "this is Dr. Marion. He's the attending pediatrician."

"Sorry we have to meet under these circumstances," I said with a smile as I shook her hand. Barefoot, wearing a peasant blouse and bell-bottom jeans, and with her long, straight brown hair parted in the middle, Jarrett's mom, who was in her early thirties, looked like a refugee from the Summer of Love. She also looked as if she could use a good night's sleep. "How are you doing?"

"Not too well," she replied. "I'm hoping someone will be able to tell me what's wrong with my son."

"We're going to try to get to the bottom of it," I said. "First, maybe you can tell me the story again from the beginning."

Without hesitation, Ms. Fox spilled out the short tale that was her son's life: After an uncomplicated pregnancy, Jarrett had been born at his parents' home in North Salem, a rural town about 50 miles north of New York City. He was the couple's second child; their daughter, Shadow, now three years old, was as healthy as a horse. Although his birth was attended only by a midwife, Jarrett was examined on his first day of life by the family's pediatrician (the only one in the area who practiced homeopathic medicine and made house calls) and declared to be in excellent health. His mother could think of nothing unusual about her son's newborn period; in her words, he had been "like any other baby."

The pediatrician had seen Jarrett again at two weeks, one month, and then at two months. He'd received his immunizations (although the family believed in homeopathic medicine and were strict vegetarians, they did understand the importance of immunizations in disease prevention), and had been growing and developing normally. Ms. Fox told me of her belief in prolonged breast-feeding: she assured me that Jarrett had eaten nothing but breast milk, adding proudly: "My daughter was exclusively breast-fed for the first two years of her life."

But this perfect infancy had ended the previous Tuesday when, according to Ms. Fox, Jarrett had awakened from his afternoon nap and simply refused to nurse. "He just wouldn't latch on to my breast," she said sadly. "Nothing I did seemed to get him interested. It was like a switch had been turned off in his brain and he wouldn't do it anymore. Just like that."

"Has he been hungry?" I asked, less certain now about the diagnosis.

"At first he was," she said. "That first day, he cried like anything. It was pathetic. But since then, he's just been kind of limp and lifeless, kind of placid, like he just didn't care anymore."

Turning my attention to the infant, I could see what Ms. Fox meant. Although a beautiful baby, Jarrett—who had an IV in his left arm and a nasogastric tube (to facilitate feeding) exiting from his left nostril (the other end passed through his pharynx, down his esophagus, and ended in his stomach)—lay limply in his hospital crib like a rag doll. His eyes did make contact with mine, but it was as if there was no sense of recognition behind those eyes. They gazed out of a face that seemed passive and expressionless.

"THIS DOESN'T SMELL like SMA," I said, shaking my head. After finishing the exam, I'd thanked Ms. Fox, told her we needed to speak with the neurologist and that we'd be back later. The team had then reassembled in the corridor, where we continued our discussion. "SMA doesn't start suddenly like this. The weakness comes on gradually over the course of a few days or weeks: the first day, the parents notice that the kid's a little floppy; the next day, he becomes a little more floppy; then he's a little more floppy the next, until finally, they find they can't get him to eat enough to keep himself going. That's when the kid comes to the hospital with dehydration and the diagnosis is made. But this story of the weakness coming on suddenly like a switch going off, that's too acute to be SMA!"

"I agree," Molly said. "It sounds almost like the kid was poisoned."

"Poisoned by what?" Eric, one of the interns, asked. "The mother's told us that the kid's eaten nothing but breast milk. If he was poisoned by something in the breast milk, the mother should have been affected also."

"Good point," I replied as a little bell of recognition began ringing in my head. "But Molly's right. The suddenness of the onset does make it sound like he has been poisoned. I think I may know what it was." Without another word, I headed back into Jarrett's room with the rest of the ward team trailing behind.

The mother, who'd been sitting on a chair at the side of Jarrett's hospital crib, rose to her feet when she saw us approach. "Sorry to bother you," I said, "but tell me again, when did you first notice this change in Jarrett?"

"Tuesday afternoon," she replied. "When he woke up from his nap. He's usually starving when he wakes up, with nursing the only thing on his mind. But that day, I couldn't get him to latch on to my breast for anything."

I nodded my head. "And your daughter. She's three?"

"Yes," Ms. Fox replied. "Shadow's three."

"Tell me, how does Shadow get along with Jarrett?"

"Oh, she's crazy about him. She loves being a big sister."

"Does she help you take care of him?" I asked.

"All the time," Ms. Fox replied with a smile. "She's always helping. She helps change his diaper, and when he spits up, she wipes him with a face cloth. She tells me that I'm her mommy and she's Jarrett's mommy."

I smiled at this also. "Since Jarrett's only breast-fed, she hasn't ever fed him, has she?"

"No, we'd never let her. But she always pretends to feed him. At mealtime, we put Jarrett's infant seat next to Shadow's chair. Sometimes she pretends to spoon food into his mouth. It's really cute and they both seem to love it."

"But as far as you know, she's never actually fed him?"

"Definitely not," Ms. Fox replied. "Either my husband or I are always at the table supervising. We'd never let Shadow put anything in the baby's mouth."

I nodded and continued: "Ms. Fox, what does Shadow eat for breakfast?"

The mother, somewhat surprised by this apparent non sequitur, answered without hesitation: "A bowl of hot oatmeal and a glass of milk. Why do you ask?"

"Does Shadow eat the oatmeal plain, or does she put sugar on it?" I asked, already knowing the answer.

As I expected she would, Ms. Fox gave me an angry look. "Dr. Marion, we do not allow sugar in our house. Sugar is poison."

"Okay, no sugar," I pushed on. "But does Shadow use anything to sweeten her oatmeal?"

"We let her use honey," she replied. "Never more than one or two teaspoons."

"Refined honey?" I asked, again knowing the answer before I asked the question.

"Of course not," the mother replied, repeating that angry look. "The refining process strips the honey of all its natural goodness. We allow only pure, unrefined honey in our house.

Everything we put into our bodies is pure and natural. That's why our family has always been so healthy."

I continued: "Ms. Fox, we have to do some tests, but I think Jarrett's going to be okay. I'm pretty sure he's got botulism."

IT WAS MS. FOX'S holier-than-thou attitude about the foods she and her family ate that tipped me off to the possibility of infant botulism—that and the suddenness with which Jarrett's symptoms began. While considering the diagnosis as I questioned her, I visualized the scenario that had undoubtedly led to the baby's sudden onset of weakness.

Early that Tuesday morning, the Foxes were all in the kitchen. Jarrett, sitting happily in his infant seat, had been placed at the table next to his big sister, who was enjoying her usual breakfast of hot oatmeal topped with a few dollops of natural honey, straight from the hive. The children's parents, although also in the kitchen, were busy with the preparation of their own breakfast, hurriedly getting ready to begin the day; as a result, they just weren't paying that much attention to their children, who after all seemed safe, content, happy, and so nearby. Suddenly, Shadow, stepping into her role as Jarrett's surrogate mother, silently offered her brother a spoonful of cereal; the infant, having never experienced the taste or feel of solid (or at least semi-solid) food in his mouth, eagerly accepted the offered spoon, and carefully rolled the strange-textured substance around in his mouth before swallowing. He smiled with satisfaction as Shadow, still in silence, finished everything in her bowl.

Later in the day, Jarrett took his usual afternoon nap. When he awakened, his mother found that, mysteriously, he could no longer latch on to her breast. As Ms. Fox continued to answer my questions, I became more convinced that this scenario (or one just like it) had occurred. It had to have; after hearing the story and seeing Jarrett, I could think of no other logical explanation.

LIKE MS. FOX, most Americans believe that when applied to foods, terms like *pure* and *natural* are synonymous with *healthy* and *nutritious*. Although this thinking may be accurate for many foods, in the case of honey, eating it in its natural state can lead to serious disease or even death. Because of the environment in which it's produced, unprocessed honey often contains spores of *Clostridium botulinum,* the bacterium that causes botulism. In most humans, the presence of these spores presents no significant problem: the environment of the stomach and intestinal tracts of older children and adults readily destroys the toxin. But in children under one year of age, infants whose intestinal tracts are still immature, the presence of the toxin, which can survive its stay in the gut unscathed, spells big trouble: after traveling through the gut's lining and entering the bloodstream, the spores are carried throughout the body, where they bind to peripheral nerves and thus prevent them from being able to carry messages from the central nervous system to the muscles. Within hours of ingesting even tiny amounts of contaminated honey, these previously healthy infants become profoundly floppy, lethargic, and placid, unable to smile or cry or suck. If the dose of spores is large enough, every muscle, including those involved in breathing, becomes paralyzed. If not recognized quickly, affected infants may simply stop breathing, suffering respiratory failure so severe that death occurs within minutes.

But if the diagnosis is made early, the prognosis for full recovery is good. Although no treatment to counteract the effect of the toxin is available, over the course of time the hold that the spores exert on the nervous system weakens and eventually wears off. If the child is supported through this period, which may last for weeks or months, if he is tube-fed, provided with oxygen, and placed on a ventilator if breathing becomes difficult, he will eventually return to the state he was in prior to the start of the disorder.

IT TOOK JARRETT FOX more than five weeks to return to his pre-poisoned state, and his road to recovery was not without complication: during the height of his illness, Jarrett was critically ill. On the afternoon of that Saturday in February, his breathing became labored, and when an analysis of his blood gases revealed a rise in carbon dioxide and a decrease in oxygen (signs of impending respiratory failure), he was transferred from the infants' unit to the intensive care unit, where he was intubated and placed on a ventilator. For weeks, he remained dependent on machines, too weak to move any of his muscles, too weak to suck or swallow, cry or smile, or breathe. He continued to be fed milk pumped from his mother's breast (she wouldn't allow him to be fed anything else) through the nasogastric tube.

When I told Ms. Fox that I believed Jarrett had botulism, she thought I was crazy. I'm sure that while I was explaining my theory of her son's illness, the one idea that passed through her mind was "I've got to get my baby out of this insane asylum as quickly as possible." But when the neurologist came by a few minutes later and agreed with me, she began to have second thoughts about her initial impression; then later, when an electromyogram (a test that measures the functioning of the muscles and nerves) revealed the presence of a profound peripheral neuropathy consistent with botulism, she, too, became positively convinced of the story I'd invented.

It took three weeks for the lab report to come back, but when it did, it confirmed the presence of the *C. botulinum* toxin not only in samples of Jarrett's serum and feces but also in a specimen taken from the jar of honey from the Foxes' pantry. Because the scenario now seemed so obvious, I urged the Foxes not to confront or blame Shadow; doing so, I argued, would do no good for Jarrett and would make the girl feel unbearably guilty. Rather, I suggested they have a talk with her, trying to get her to understand that she should never put anything into her little brother's mouth.

Then in early March, Jarrett's nurse noted what appeared to be a flicker of movement in his left leg. Although it was initially so subtle that she thought she'd only imagined it, in the hours that followed more movements occurred. Slowly, the toxin was losing its control over Jarrett's peripheral nervous system. His muscles were coming back to life.

In the next few days, he was gradually weaned off the ventilator and ultimately extubated. Tentatively, he began eating on his own again, first from a syringe, then from a bottle, and finally, more than a month after he'd entered the hospital, directly from his mother's breast. With the help of our physical and occupational therapists, his muscles were exercised and strengthened; he was discharged to home at the beginning of April, essentially back to his old self.

Ms. Fox continued to preach that the natural foods that filled the Foxes' pantry were the only way to maintain good health. By the time Jarrett left the hospital, however, she was able to accept the fact that the pure, natural honey she had demanded her family use had been the cause of her son's serious illness.

CHAPTER 9

The Christmas Present

TELLING PARENTS THAT their child has a genetic disease is definitely the worst part of my job. Often painful, always distressing, it's unfortunately something we clinical geneticists can't avoid: so many of the conditions with which we deal have such terrible prognoses. In these situations we are forced to act as judge and jury. Because he is affected with a disorder, we have found the child guilty, and it's our role to condemn him to death and his family to a lifetime of grief. In most cases, once the diagnosis has been confirmed and the news delivered, we're helpless to do anything to avert the predetermined outcome. We can't fix the child's problem, we often can't even significantly alter the course of his illness. At best, in an attempt to make his existence as acceptable as possible, all we can really hope to do is orchestrate some of the events of the child's and the family's life.

That's what happened the first time I saw the Sweeneys.

It was the Friday before Christmas, and the Garwood Children's Rehabilitation Hospital in Westchester County had that feeling of forced festivity that tends to envelop children's hospitals during the holiday season. It seemed as if every last inch of the place was covered with tinsel and blinking lights, garishly decorated evergreens, and giant menorahs. In spite of all these carefully arranged, colorful, and cheerful decorations, a feeling of helplessness and hopelessness still hung in the air.

Amy McDonald, a second-year fellow in genetics, and I were standing in the hallway talking with Ben Sontag, the executive director of Garwood, when we first saw the Sweeneys: mother, father, and son were rapidly walking down the hall toward the outpatient department. From my vantage point, I could only see the boy in profile; Amy was able to see him straight on. Each of us saw the child for no more than a few seconds, clutching the hands of his parents for support, as he walked past us. But that brief glimpse was enough: his coarse facial features, his thick, clawlike hands, and his stiff hunched gait told us more than either the fellow or I needed to know. I looked at Amy, she looked at me, and our jaws dropped.

"What's wrong?" Ben asked, noticing the change in our demeanor.

"That boy . . . ," Amy began.

"What about him?" Ben asked, looking down the hall, probably taking notice of the family for the first time.

"He's got a mucopolysaccharidosis," I replied.

"I'm sure he does," Ben said. "What's a mucopolysaccharidosis?"

"A lysosomal storage disease," Amy responded. "One of a

group of disorders that usually causes degeneration of the central nervous system and early death."

"You can tell all that just by seeing the boy pass in the hall for a few seconds?" Ben asked.

"Ben, if we couldn't tell all that just by seeing him pass in the hall, we wouldn't deserve to be your genetics consultants," I replied.

"It looks to me like he probably has Hunter syndrome," Amy added.

"Hunter syndrome I know about," Ben said. "At least I know enough to know that Hunter syndrome is not a good thing to have."

Amy and I nodded. "We'd better go find out why that kid's here," I said.

By this point the family had disappeared around the corner that led to the outpatient department. Amy and I followed down the hall after them and, seeing that the parents had settled themselves in the waiting area while the boy had begun to attack the well-stocked toy chest, we entered the reception station.

"Who's that kid?" I asked Joanne, the clerk.

"Thomas Sweeney," Joanne replied. "Your first patient of the afternoon."

After pulling the boy's chart from the To Be Seen basket, I began riffling through it. I found the Genetics Consultation Request Form, and my heart sank as I read it. "A three-year-old who was referred for evaluation by Eileen Woods, the audiologist," I mumbled in Amy's direction. "He has hearing loss and global developmental delay."

"Does it say anything about his having Hunter syndrome?" Amy asked.

I turned the pages of the chart. Results of an audiogram revealed that the boy had mild to moderate conductive hearing loss. A note from Eileen briefly outlined the boy's history: a year before, he'd been able to say a half dozen words; more recently, not only had he not gained any new words or started putting them together in sentences, but he'd apparently regressed, losing all ability to communicate verbally. Except for this note and some insurance information, the chart was empty. "No, no diagnosis listed," I said to Amy. "We'd better go talk to Eileen."

We found the audiologist sitting in her office, doing some paperwork. "Thomas Sweeney's here to see us," I said, taking a seat across from Eileen's desk. "Looking at him, we think he might have Hunter syndrome or one of the other mucopolysaccharidoses. Do you know if anyone's raised this possibility with the parents in the past?"

The audiologist shook her head. "Apparently not," she replied. "I saw him for the first time a couple of weeks ago. His parents made the appointment themselves because Tommy's speech is so delayed. They've been worried about him for over a year, but their pediatrician has been blowing them off, telling them that he's just a little slow in getting started and that he'll eventually catch up."

"Terrific," Amy interrupted. "That's very helpful."

"The parents knew Tommy was more than just a little slow," Eileen continued, "and since they weren't getting any help from their doctor, they finally decided to take matters into their own hands. When I saw him, I knew he had something, but I wasn't sure what it was."

"How did you get them to make an appointment to see us?" I asked.

"That was easy. Since the audiogram showed that he had significant hearing loss, I told them that sometimes these kinds of problems were inherited, and that it might be a good idea for Tommy to see a geneticist. It didn't take a lot to convince them; the mom told me that they've put off having more children until they get an answer about what's causing Tommy's problem. They're very nice people, and they're scared to death."

"They have good reason to be," I said. "You know what happens to kids with Hunter syndrome?"

Eileen nodded her head. An experienced audiologist, she had worked at Garwood long enough to have cared for a few children and adolescents with various forms of mucopolysaccharidoses. Over the years, she'd carefully and methodically documented the inevitable slow, steady deterioration of their speech and hearing.

"Do you have any feel for how they're going to take this news?" Amy asked.

The audiologist hesitated for only a few seconds. "They're going to be devastated," she said.

I nodded, and Amy and I left her office.

BECAUSE IT WAS the Friday of a holiday weekend, most everyone at Garwood had planned to leave work early in an attempt to get a jump on the traffic. Before starting with the Sweeneys, I wanted to make sure that all the tests needed to confirm the suspected diagnosis could be performed. Amy and I went into our office, located in the hospital's administrative suite, and started making phone calls. I called the X-ray tech, to see if she'd be able to do a skeletal survey in about an hour, while Amy called the lab to make sure they'd be open to draw the blood, collect the urine, and box all the specimens so they could be mailed to our reference lab. In neither case were the people on the other end of the phone exactly overjoyed at the prospects of having to deal with a child with a mucopolysaccharidosis that afternoon. But both reluctantly agreed that if we got the patient to them by three, they'd do what needed to be done.

After hanging up the phone, I sat back in my desk chair and sighed. "I really hate this part," I said sadly to Amy. "I hate having to tell them. But we've got to do it, so we might as well get it over with."

As I was beginning to rise, Amy said, "Bob, are you sure you want to do this?"

"No, I'm pretty sure I don't want to do this," I said, sitting back in my chair. "But what choice do we have?"

"Look, it's three days before Christmas. If this boy has Hunter syndrome, he's had it for three years, right?"

"Right," I replied.

"And if he's had it for three years, isn't he also likely to still have it next week and the week after that?"

I nodded.

"Right," Amy continued. "Christmas is going to be hard enough for these people as it is. Look at what they're going through. They know something's wrong with their only child, something that's preventing him from being able to speak. It's got to be frustrating for them, but at least without a name for the condition or a prognosis, they still can hold on to some hope. I'm sure that, deep down, they both believe that whatever's wrong can be fixed with either medication or surgery, or that it might even resolve on its own. Do you agree?"

I again nodded.

Amy continued: "Now think of what Christmas will be like if we tell them that their son has an incurable neurodegenerative disease that not only will prevent him from ever being able to communicate but will also wind up killing him by the time he's 20."

I paused to think about Amy's words. "You're absolutely right," I finally responded. "Telling them today would destroy whatever joy they might have had over the next week."

"It would be different if we had some treatment to offer, or if there was a pregnancy involved," Amy went on. "But there is no magic pill, and Eileen just told us that they're holding off having more children until they know for sure exactly what's wrong with the boy. Making the diagnosis today, next week, or even next month won't change anything."

I continued to nod. "There's only one problem," I said. "They're already here for their appointment. I don't feel comfortable seeing them and not telling them what we think."

The office remained silent as both Amy and I thought through this problem, trying to come up with a solution. Finally, reaching for the phone, I broke the silence: "I'm just going to have to lie," I said. As I dialed the number of the outpatient department's reception station, I added, "Now, Amy,

I want you to understand, I'm not encouraging or condoning this kind of behavior. But, occasionally, not telling the truth may be in the best interest of the patient and his family."

After two rings, the clerk picked up the phone. "Joanne," I said, trying to sound as pained as possible, "this is Bob Marion. I'm sorry to do this. I know I have a patient waiting out there, but I've developed a terrible migraine headache. I have to take some medication and lie down for a while. Would you apologize to them for me and reschedule them for the first Friday in January?"

When I emerged from my office a half hour later, miraculously cured of my devastating headache and ready to see my next patient, the Sweeneys were gone. Amy and I saw the remainder of the patients scheduled for the genetics clinic that afternoon. When we left a nearly deserted Garwood, I was still thinking about the Sweeneys, still turning over in my mind whether we'd truly done the right thing.

DURING THE SWEENEYS' visit in early January, Amy and I finally had to face telling them our concerns. As we'd expected, the session was difficult. The couple, understanding all too well what we were saying, at first denied that Tommy had anything worse than just some mild hearing loss; but ultimately, faced with all the evidence we presented, they came to accept our conclusion. As they held hands, both crying softly, we told them that no matter what the workup showed, regardless of whether Tommy had Hunter syndrome, one of the other mucopolysaccharidoses, some other condition, or nothing at all, we'd be there for them, always available to offer information and advice, to follow their son during the years to come, and just to talk.

We did a complete evaluation of Tommy that afternoon. X-rays of the boy's bones showed that he had dysostosis multiplex, the typical appearance seen in the mucopolysaccharidoses; a urine sample showed equal but markedly elevated excretion of the chemicals dermatan sulfate and heparan sulfate; and an assay of iduronate sulfatase performed on a blood sample revealed a complete absence of enzyme activity; all of these confirmed the diagnosis of Hunter syndrome.

It's been more than a month now since I called Mr. Sweeney's office to tell him that the lab tests had confirmed what we all already knew. The boy, who almost immediately began a course of rigorous physical, occupational, and speech therapy, has already shown some improvement in his motor skills, but his lack of speech continues unchanged. I check in with Tommy's mother and father at least once a week, trying to ensure in my own mind that they're weathering this emotional storm. They seem to be doing as well as can be expected. Mrs. Sweeney told me last week that although falling asleep at night continues to be difficult, she and her husband have finally achieved something of a milestone: they've been able to make it through the day without crying.

While at Garwood for clinic yesterday, I spoke with Mr. Sweeney. We were talking about how life had changed for the family since Tommy's diagnosis was confirmed, and, for the first time, we discussed Christmas.

"You can't imagine how perfect that day was," Mr. Sweeney said. "Our house was filled with laughter and happiness. Our parents came for dinner, we exchanged presents, and of course, as the only grandchild on either side, Tommy was the center of attention. When I think of what's happened since then, I can't believe how happy we all were. I'll always remember that last Christmas; it was the last time that our world seemed anything like normal."

After a few minutes, we said goodbye, and after hanging up, I just sat in my office chair, thinking. I've turned over in my mind many times since that late December day whether or not telling that lie was the right thing to do. Though, in general, it's difficult to justify lying to patients, I've decided that in some situations, in some circumstances, it may be acceptable. Holding back the news from the Sweeneys on that Friday before Christmas was one of those justifiable situations; by not seeing the family, Amy and I made sure that they'd have one last memorable holiday before their lives were irretrievably changed. That lie was our Christmas present to the Sweeneys.

Postscript

PUBLISHED IN THE *American Journal of Medical Genetics* in 1996, my essay about Thomas Sweeney and his family evoked a sizable response. Apparently, it hit a nerve in the clinical genetics community. Many of us, faced regularly with receiving news of an abnormality in a prenatal diagnosis specimen from the lab on a Friday afternoon or on the eve of a holiday, never really feel comfortable with the decision about whether to inform the family or wait. On the one hand, because there's no chance for any intervention over the weekend or during the holiday, it seems like cruel and unusual punishment to force people to live with the knowledge for three or four days. On the other hand, it could be argued that such reasoning is paternalistic, that the family members, not the geneticist, should be the ones making this decision.

Of the letters that were received by the journal, the most troubling to me came from Alan Donnenfeld, a geneticist in Philadelphia, who recounted the following story:

A woman had undergone an amniocentesis because of advanced maternal age shortly before Christmas. The results were communicated to us on Christmas Eve and indicated that the fetus was affected with Down syndrome. We discussed this case at length amongst our genetic staff and tried to decide whether it would be best to call the patient that evening or wait until the day after Christmas. The impression from the genetic counselor who met with this couple . . . was extremely important in rendering our decision. We concluded, similarly to Dr. Marion, that informing the family on Christmas Eve would be devastating and of no potential benefit since we could not meet and provide genetic counseling the following day (as is our custom when we inform patients of an abnormal prenatal result). We thought that telling them on Christmas Eve would destroy their holiday and lead to no potential benefit. We called the patient the day after Christmas. She was devastated. Then she said something which made us cringe, "I wish I had known before Christmas. Yesterday, at a family gathering with all my dearest relatives, I announced that I was going to have a baby. If I had only known this information beforehand, I would not have told anyone."

Dr. Donnenfeld ended his letter by noting, "Sometimes, despite the best of our intentions, decisions designed to spare patients from experiencing unnecessary grief, lead to unfortunate consequences."[1]

It's a tough path to walk. On the one hand, we want to do what's best for our patients and their families; on the other hand, we don't want to be paternalistic, making decisions that we think are in our patients' best interest without any input from them. Being rigid, taking one tack (such as always immediately informing the family of results or of our impression) may be the easiest position to assume; however, doing this may also cause difficulties for the family. Therefore, I think I'll continue doing what I've always done—that is, address each case individually, taking what I know about the family into account, making the decision I think is best. It may be paternalistic, but in most cases this approach seems to work.

Since Tommy Sweeney was diagnosed, there has been a breakthrough in the treatment of Hunter syndrome, but that breakthrough has itself led to some controversy. In 2006, the U.S. Food and Drug Administration approved the use of Elaprase (a form of the enzyme iduronate sulfatase) for individuals with Hunter syndrome. The drug has been shown to improve cardiovascular, pulmonary, and orthopedic functioning of men and boys with the disease. (Unlike the other mucopolysaccharidoses, all of which are autosomal recessively inherited, Hunter syndrome is X-linked recessive, passed from unaffected mothers to their sons, each of whom has a 50 percent chance of being affected; thus, virtually all individuals with Hunter syndrome are male.) However, the inability of Elaprase to cross the blood-brain barrier—the membranous structure that protects the brain from chemicals circulating in the bloodstream—prevents it from having any effect on the central nervous system of these individuals. Thus, even with treatment, males with Hunter syndrome continue to experience the neurologic deterioration that characterizes the disorder. Because of this, Tommy's parents decided not to use Elaprase on their son, reasoning that the benefit was not worth the weekly intravenous infusions required.

I continued to follow Tommy Sweeney at Garwood until his family relocated to Louisiana when the boy was four. Although I'm no longer his doctor, I still get Christmas cards from the family every year. Each card is accompanied by a picture of Tommy, photographs that, through the years, have documented the slow, steady downhill course this devastating disease has taken on his mind and his body. And every December, when I get the Sweeneys' card, I'm always struck by how ironic it is that these cards celebrate Christmas, that holiday that will cause me to always remember Tommy and his parents.

THE CHRISTMAS SEASON has always been difficult for me. Around the end of one year and the start of the next, parents like the Sweeneys often take stock of their lives; they realize that the clock is ticking, that their child is getting worse and that there probably won't be that many festive occasions remaining before the inevitable occurs. So, over the years, I've learned to try to find ways to make the holidays more joyous for my patients. Sometimes a patient finds a way to make the season more joyous for me. That happened during my internship, when I took care of Andre Watson.

In December of that year, the director of our training program decided to try an experiment. To give us quality time with our loved ones, instead of the usual every-third-night-on-call that characterized the rest of the year, the chief resident assigned us to work two consecutive nights. We were scheduled to work Christmas Eve and Christmas Day, New Year's Eve and New Year's Day, or two of the days in between. By so doing, each intern would manage to get a four-day mini-holiday.

It was a good idea, and having those four days in a row off in the middle of our internship year was terrific for our morale, but the price we had to pay was exceedingly high: each of us would have to spend more than 50 consecutive hours working in the hospital without relief. During that month, I was rotating on Children's 2, the pediatric infectious disease floor. When the December on-call schedule was posted at the end of November, I found my name aside the dates December 24 and December 25.

That year, December 24 fell on a Tuesday. As usual, I got to work at 7:00 A.M. and began the routine tasks interns perform on regular weekday mornings. After checking on each of my patients (I had six at the start of the day), I went on work rounds with the rest of our ward team. At 10:00 A.M., Dr. Mann, our attending physician, came to do rounds, which ran until about noon. After these formal activities ended, the two other interns who were working on the floor that month finished their work as quickly as they could and signed out to me. It being Christmas Eve, they both had plans and wanted to get out of the hospital as early as possible.

So by 3:30 that afternoon, I was essentially alone. The other interns were gone, the medical students were on vacation, and the resident who was on call with me was also covering three other wards. He came to check in only twice that evening. That was it: just me, two nurses who would have much rather been home celebrating with their families, and about a dozen patients, children who, despite our best efforts to get them out of the hospital for the holiday, were just too sick to be discharged.

It would be difficult to find anything sadder than a pediatric ward on Christmas Eve. During the preceding days, the ward clerk and some kindly volunteers had spent hours covering the walls of the unit with decorations. Near the nurses' station, there was a plastic tree and a large electric menorah. But in spite of all these cheerful dressings, it still didn't feel right. Some of the children on the ward that night were infants, too young to realize how rotten a deal they'd gotten. But the others, sick though they were, knew that this was not how Christmas was supposed to be spent.

At least for most of the kids, Christmas Eve was improved by the fact that their families had come to spend the holiday with them, but like me, Andre Watson was all alone that night. Andre, an eight-year-old from Detroit, had been put on a plane by his mother so that he could come to Boston the Friday before to visit his aunt and her family for the holidays. He'd developed a high fever on Saturday, and he'd become nearly comatose by

Sunday morning. Terrified that he was going to die, his aunt had brought him to our emergency room, where a spinal tap confirmed what the ER doc had suspected: the boy had bacterial meningitis, a serious, potentially deadly infection of the fluid that bathes the brain. An IV was started, massive doses of antibiotics were pushed into his vein, and Andre was admitted for careful monitoring and completion of the course of antibiotics.

Although Andre had been critically ill when he'd come up to our floor, in the 48 hours that had passed, his condition had significantly improved. On Monday, he'd awakened from his coma; that night, his temperature had returned to normal for the first time in two days. By Tuesday afternoon, although he was still pretty sick, he'd been alert enough to know that it was Christmas Eve, that he was alone in a strange city, and that he was terrified.

I understood from the start that in order to survive two straight nights on call, I was going to have to pace myself. I would need to get my work done and get to sleep as early as possible. At around six o'clock on Tuesday evening, I got an admission: a four-month-old girl with pneumonia. It took me about two hours to get that baby—who was febrile, breathing rapidly, and in need of supplemental oxygen but otherwise not very sick—worked up and settled in. At around eight o'clock, I did evening rounds. My plan was to check all 13 patients on the floor and get done any scut that needed doing. According to my plan, if there were no screw-ups, I'd make it into the bed in the on-call room by ten at the latest.

As the sickest patient on the floor, Andre had been placed in the room at the end of the hall closest to the nurses' station.

Since I started rounds at the other end of the ward, he was the last patient I checked on that night. Because his condition was contagious, Andre had been placed alone, though his room had two beds. Upon entering, I found the boy lying in bed, crying to himself. "What's wrong?" I asked as I checked his vital signs on the bedside clipboard.

At first, he didn't say anything; he just continued to cry. I put down the clipboard and looked directly at him. "What's wrong?" I asked again. "Is anything bothering you?"

He shook his head.

"Does it hurt where they stuck the needle in your back?"

He shook his head again.

"Does your head hurt?"

Again that shake.

"Is it because it's Christmas?"

His crying increased.

"I know, I know," I said, patting him on the shoulder. "It's Christmas Eve, you're sick, you're in the hospital, and you're all alone. Is that it?"

He nodded.

"Is your aunt coming?" I asked.

Andre shook his head and continued to cry. (I found out later that one of Andre's cousins was home in bed with the flu. Figuring that Andre would be well cared for by the hospital's staff, his aunt chose to remain home with her sick daughter, who otherwise would have had no one to care for her.)

I sighed. "Well, I know how you're feeling. At least a little. I'm all alone here, too. Do you think it would help if you could speak to your mother?"

For the first time, the boy looked up at me. He nodded.

Although Andre's room had a phone, he couldn't make long-distance calls. And because he was still contagious enough to be confined to his room, getting him to the nurses' station, where long-distance service was available, was problematic. So, assuring him I'd be right back, I went out to the clerk's desk and, after finding his home phone number in the chart, called his mother in Detroit. I explained that although Andre was feeling better, he was terribly sad. I told her the only thing that would cheer him up was hearing her voice. She said she'd call right away.

By the time I got back to his room, Andre was cradling the receiver to his ear. His tears were gone and he was smiling. I heard him tell his mother how much he missed her.

I don't know exactly how long they talked. After seeing that my treatment had cured his problem, at least temporarily, I left the room, going back to get my work done. Half an hour later, having completed the scut work that had been left over from earlier in the day, I stopped back in Andre's room on my way to the on-call room. The boy was sitting up in bed, watching a Christmas special on TV. "Do you feel better?" I asked.

He nodded.

"Good," I said. "I'm going off to try to get some sleep now. If you need anything, just ask the nurse and she'll come get me. Okay?"

He shook his head.

"What's wrong?" I asked.

"My mother said . . . she said that maybe if I asked you, you might be able to stay in my room with me. In that bed . . ." He pointed to the room's second bed.

"You want me to sleep in your room?" I asked.

He nodded and I smiled.

"Okay. It is Christmas Eve, and we're both alone here. Okay, I'll sleep in here. But we've got to go to bed right now. You've got to turn off the TV."

While Andre got ready to go to sleep, I walked out to the nurses' station and told the nurses that if they needed me, I'd be sleeping in Andre's room. By the time I got back, the television and room lights had been turned off. In another couple of minutes, after I'd taken off my shoes and gotten into the spare bed, Andre's breathing had settled into a regular, undisturbed pattern. I nodded off sometime after that.

That night, mercifully, the nurses awakened me only once. At 4:00 A.M., the beautiful IV I'd placed in the arm of the newly admitted four-month-old with pneumonia infiltrated just before her next dose of antibiotics was due. I can't say restarting it was too much of an ordeal, though. By that point in the year, I'd become pretty proficient at putting in IVs, and despite the infant's screaming and squirming, I managed to get another line started on the very first try. After completing the job, I got back into the second bed in Andre's room, and slept undisturbed until seven the next morning.

Andre was still sound asleep when I crept out of my bed. I noticed his eyes opening as, having picked up my clipboard, my stethoscope, and my beeper, I tried to sneak silently out of the room.

After taking a shower and changing into a fresh set of scrubs in the interns' on-call room, I was back on the floor by 7:30. During the half hour I'd been gone, the place had come to life. The parents who'd come to spend the holiday with their children had brought along Christmas presents, and torn wrapping paper, dolls, and battery-operated mechanical toys were everywhere. For the first time, the place actually started to feel like it was a holiday.

The resident who was covering me was sitting in the nurses' station, taking all this in. We began work rounds; together, we walked to the end of the hall, turned, and worked our way back. We stopped outside each room, checked the vital-sign sheets, briefly examined each child, then made plans for the day. On a sheet of paper attached to the top of my clipboard, I generated a fresh scut list that would have to be completed that morning.

By the time we made it to Andre's room, the boy was dressed and sitting up on his bed. The night before, I'd told him that in the morning his isolation would officially be lifted and he'd be allowed to leave his room and mingle with the other patients, and he was raring to go. When we gave him the news that he was cleared, he got up and headed straight for the ward's playroom, pushing his IV pole in front of him.

For me, Christmas was busier than I expected. I spent the whole day working, not even getting the chance to watch when Santa Claus (played by one of the critical care attending physicians) came ho-ho-ho-ing onto Children's 2 to distribute presents. After I finished my scut and wrote a brief progress note on each patient, the admissions started rolling in. During the day, I got four new patients, including one critically ill child, a four-year-old who, like Andre, had been diagnosed in the emergency room with bacterial meningitis. Getting these new patients settled, starting IVs, sending off blood work, and writing nursing orders and admission notes took most of the day. By 8:00 P.M., as I sat in the nurses' station working on the last of the admission notes, I was fighting to keep my eyes open. Unfortunately, I lost the battle.

For the first time that year, I actually fell asleep sitting up, while writing on a chart. My head came to rest on my folded hands and I just started snoring. When I awoke something like an hour later, I was surprised to find that a blanket had been thrown around my shoulders. Wiping the sleep from my eyes, I saw Andre standing about ten feet away. "Are you okay?" I asked.

"Yeah, I'm fine, Dr. Bob. Look what Santa brought me." He held up a huge magic set.

"Andre the Magnificent," I said with a smile.

"Are you okay, Dr. Bob? Don't you ever get to leave the hospital?"

I laughed. "I've got to stay all night again tonight. I'll be going home tomorrow. I guess I fell asleep."

"I know," Andre replied. "You were sitting there, snoring real loud! It sounded like someone was sawing wood. I put that blanket on you."

"That was a really nice thing to do, Andre. Thank you."

"I thought you were going to get cold."

After finishing the admission note on which I'd been working when I fell asleep, I sluggishly rose and trudged down the hall, making evening rounds once again before going off to sleep. Worried, I guess, that I might fall asleep in the middle of the hall, Andre walked alongside, carrying my clipboard, trying to help me as much as he could. When we were finished,

I walked him back into his room. "I'm going to the on-call room to get some sleep now," I said.

"Can't you sleep in here again tonight?" he asked.

Smiling, I said, "I guess so," and fell back into the room's spare bed. "You don't think my snoring will keep you up?"

"It didn't last night," Andre replied.

On Christmas night, I fell asleep before Andre did. The nurses tortured me most of that night, awakening me six times. I finally got up for good at 6:30 on the morning of December 26. After taking another shower and changing into yet another set of clean scrubs, I sat in the nurses' station, waiting for the rest of the team to arrive. I was never so happy to see my fellow interns!

During work rounds that morning, we redistributed the patients. I wound up being the primary doctor for only four of them. I made sure that one of my patients was Andre Watson. Andre and I had become pals—we'd looked out for each other, we'd become a team, and I didn't want to break that team up.

That morning, I somehow managed to make it through both work rounds and attending rounds. I wrote notes on my patients and, by 2:00 P.M., was ready to sign out to the intern who was on call that night. Before leaving, I made sure to say goodbye to Andre, who was busy with the magic kit the critical care Santa had given him.

"You're finally going home?" he asked.

"Finally going home," I repeated. "I've been here for 55 hours straight. It's time to go get some quality sleep. I'll see you tomorrow."

Before I left, the boy told me to drive carefully.

ANDRE REMAINED IN the hospital for another week, finishing off his course of intravenous antibiotics. On January 3, I discharged him to his mother, who'd flown out from Detroit to pick him up and take him home. I hugged the boy before he left, and told his mother to take good care of him.

"Thank you for making me better, Dr. Bob," he said as he and his mom headed for the ward's door.

"Thank you for making Christmas a little merrier for me," I said back to him.

I've never seen Andre again. But every Christmas, I think of him . . . Andre the Magnificent. And I'm grateful for the gift of companionship he gave me during that long two-day ordeal.

CHAPTER 10

Erin, Before I Knew Her

I USUALLY FIRST MEET my patients and their families during times of crisis. As was the case with the Sweeneys, a referral is made because a genetic problem is suspected in a young child. I see the child, make a diagnosis, inform the parents of that diagnosis, and by so doing propel the family's world into turmoil. As I mentioned before, it's as if I really have two patients: the child with the disease and his or her family. My role in looking after the child is usually fairly straightforward; my role with the other patient, however, is less so. Hoping to minimize the damage to the family members, attempting to ease their suffering, I try to provide them with as much support as I can, offering ongoing counseling and anticipatory guidance. Eventually, my second patient's need for attention diminishes. Once the news has been digested and accepted, the crisis passes; loved ones put their lives back in order as best they can. But life never returns to what had been normal; having a child with a chronic disease changes most families irrevocably.

But it was well after this initial crisis had passed that I met the Wood family for the first time. Although I've come to know these people fairly well in the years that have passed since that first visit, it wasn't until I'd been working with them for six years that I came to understand a little better what really makes them tick.

We first met when Erin was 13 years old. Her father had been transferred to New York and the family—composed of Erin, her parents, and her older brother—had relocated to Connecticut from the suburb of Detroit, Michigan, where they'd lived since well before Erin's birth. In trying to find a new health care provider for her daughter, Mrs. Wood had called Garwood Children's Hospital in an attempt to find out if any of the doctors on staff even knew what Sanfilippo syndrome type B was. The clerk in the outpatient department had scheduled an appointment for the girl to see me the following week.

I clearly remember that first visit. When I called them into my office, Erin, crouched slightly and holding tightly to her mother's hand for support, plodded along slowly and clumsily from the waiting area, her gait wide-based and unsure, like a bear stumbling around after being prematurely awakened from hibernation. During the brief journey from the waiting area into the office and during the entire time I took the history from her mother, Erin kept her large head down, her chin resting on her chest, as if she didn't possess the muscular strength to support its weight. At no time did Erin say a word, utter a sound, or make any effort to communicate. Although she was smaller than would be expected for a girl of her age, the acne that dotted her face told me that she had entered puberty, a fact that Mrs. Wood soon confirmed.

In my office, Mrs. Wood unraveled the basic story of her daughter's life. Completely normal at birth, Erin had seemed fine during her first year of life. Then, sometime after her first birthday, the Woods had noticed some disturbing things about their daughter. Her development, though technically on target, seemed slower than their son's had been. And although her mother described her as a "good baby," the Woods noticed early on that Erin was exquisitely sensitive to sound, reacting violently to the slamming of a door, the ringing of the telephone, the honking of a car horn. Although they brought these and other concerns to the attention of their pediatrician, he repeatedly reassured them that Erin was fine, that these so-called problems were normal aspects of early childhood development, and that he was certain that their concerns would fade into memories as the months went by.

But as time passed, rather than being reassured by their pediatrician's words, the Woods grew more and more concerned about their daughter. Although Erin had been able to say about a dozen words at a year of age, her vocabulary had increased very little during her second year of life. At two years (an age at which their son had had a repertory of more than 100 words and had begun to form sentences), Erin had a total of only about 30 words, which she repeated regularly and meaningfully. Unsure of what any of this might mean, the couple continued seeing their regular doctor, hoping that his intuition was correct. But in their hearts, Mrs. Wood told me, both she and her husband had become convinced that there was something wrong with their daughter.

Their fears were finally confirmed when Erin was four years old. One morning the girl developed a high fever. Finding that their regular pediatrician was on vacation, the mother brought Erin to see the physician who was covering. That pediatrician took one look at the little girl, sighed, and began questioning Mrs. Wood about her daughter's development. "She knew right away," Mrs. Wood told me.

In addition to a prescription for amoxicillin to treat the ear infection that had caused the fever, Mrs. Wood was given a referral to a geneticist. Once that referral was made, the remainder of the story passed lightning fast: the tests ordered by the geneticist revealed that Erin's urine contained massive amounts of heparan sulfate; an assay of a blood sample showed a marked deficiency of the enzyme N-acetyl-alpha-glucosaminidase in the girl's white blood cells. Less than two weeks after their first visit to his office, the geneticist told the couple that their daughter had a condition called Sanfilippo syndrome. Unfortunately, it was also his job to explain to them precisely what Erin's future was likely to hold.

LIKE THE HUNTER SYNDROME that caused the slow, steady deterioration in Tommy Sweeney, Sanfilippo syndrome is one of the mucopolysaccharidoses, a family of inherited disorders in which, because of the deficiency of a naturally occurring enzyme, the cells of the body can't break down and dispose of a group of complex chemicals called glycoaminoglycans (GAGs), formerly called mucopolysaccharides. As in Hunter syndrome, the result is that these chemicals build up in the bloodstream and are then deposited in the organs of the body. The storage of GAGs in the central nervous system leads to a plateauing of development and then a steady deterioration of neurologic functioning. At its end stage, as in Alzheimer's disease at the other end of life, it is as if the child with Sanfilippo syndrome has ceased to exist; her lungs still exchange air, her heart still beats, but the mind that made her a unique individual has essentially vanished.

As mentioned earlier, in reference to Tommy Sweeney, a lot of progress has been made over the past few years in treating some of the mucopolysaccharidoses. We've gained the ability to replace the enzyme that is missing in the bloodstream of individuals with some forms of mucopolysaccharidoses, effectively reversing the downhill course. But as is the case in Hunter syndrome, because the enzyme that is replaced through intravenous infusion cannot cross the blood-brain barrier, those affected with Sanfilippo syndrome do not benefit from these treatments and their central nervous systems continue to deteriorate. So, even today, when we confirm the diagnosis of Sanfilippo syndrome in a young child, the counseling we give the family is no different from that which the Wood family received from the geneticist in Detroit when Erin was four: the prognosis is bleak.

SITTING IN MY OFFICE at Garwood that first time we met, Mrs. Wood told me that nearly all of the predictions made by the geneticist in Detroit had come true. Over time, Erin had slowly lost her ability to communicate with the outside world.

By age five, no longer able to repeat the words she'd mastered earlier in life, she was able to tell her parents of her needs and wants only by grunting and pointing. At eight, the grunting stopped. By ten, she no longer pointed. And according to her mother, at the time I first met her, Erin was "locked in," existing but able to do little else. She ate and drank when food and water were placed in her mouth; she wet and soiled her diapers; the year before, she'd begun menstruating and now had a menstrual period every month or so. But Erin had lost the use of the most important part of her brain. And once she had surrendered the use of these important neurons to this terrible disease, there would be no way that anyone would ever be able to restore this function.

My physical examination of Erin pretty much confirmed all this. As I made my way through the exam, checking her from top to bottom, the girl made no signal to me that she was present in the room. She spoke no words, nor did she make an attempt to grunt; she didn't gesture or point or make any eye contact. All through the time I spent with her, I had the sense that I was examining a manikin.

But except for this lack of ability to interact, Erin seemed to be in good health. Toward the end of that first visit, I outlined a plan of management for Mrs. Wood: I scheduled appointments for Erin to see the cardiologist, ophthalmologist, and physiatrist for baseline evaluations. I made sure the family had all the equipment they needed to care for Erin comfortably at home. Finally, we talked about how the family was functioning. Although Mrs. Wood told me they were all fine, I could tell from her words and see in her eyes that she, at least, was depressed.

When I suggested that she might benefit from talking with one of Garwood's psychologists who was experienced in caring for families of children with chronic diseases, she jumped at the opportunity. And finally, I scheduled an appointment for Erin to come back to see me after all of this was completed. I knew there was little I would be able to do to help Erin; I was more concerned about Mrs. Wood and the rest of her family.

AS THE YEARS PASSED, Erin and her mother came to see me every six months. I would spend the first part of each visit talking with Mrs. Wood about Erin's recent health issues; then I'd do a quick physical exam. The bulk of the visit would be spent talking about how the family was holding up and coping.

Through the years after the Woods' first visit, Erin remained healthy, but there was an undeniable, steady deterioration in her functioning. Two years after her first visit to Garwood, the girl required the use of a walker for support when ambulating. One year later, she came in a wheelchair. "At home, she walks most of the time," Mrs. Wood explained to me during that visit. "We only use the chair when she has to walk long distances, like from the parking lot to the outpatient department." Sometime after that visit, though, Erin became dependent on the wheelchair; it had become her only means of transport.

And there was other deterioration as well. No longer able to hold her head up independently, Erin by this time had to be positioned in her wheelchair using specially designed straps and belts. She had trouble handling her own secretions and drooled excessively, causing the skin around her mouth to break down and become infected. Feeding her also became difficult; now that she was less willing to chew and swallow solid foods on her own, the family sometimes had to resort to the use of a feeding tube, passed through the girl's nose and threaded into her stomach, in order to provide her with enough calories to maintain her weight.

Through all those years, the Woods remained steadfastly committed to caring for Erin in their home. Even though her care was so difficult and the rewards appeared to be so meager, the couple would not even consider placing their daughter in a chronic care facility. "She's our burden," Mrs. Wood told me when I brought up the topic during the girl's visits to Garwood. "Erin is our child, our responsibility, and we'll do everything we can to make her comfortable. She'll stay at home with us until the end."

From the Erin Wood that I had come to know over the previous six years, I found her mother's position difficult to understand. Spending virtually all of one's time changing diapers, lugging nearly 100 pounds of essentially dead weight from bed to wheelchair and back again, forcing food down an unresponsive gullet, bathing skin irritated by perpetual drooling, caring for a person who has seemingly ceased to be a person, and getting what appears to be nothing in return seems like a senseless way to live one's life. But one day, Mrs. Wood told me a story that made me understand why the family was so adamant about their home care.

THIS PARTICULAR VISIT was slightly unusual. Accompanying me that day was a fourth-year medical school student who was doing an elective in medical genetics. In an attempt to teach her about my specialty, knowing she might never again see a patient with Sanfilippo syndrome, I spent the first part of my visit with Mrs. Wood reviewing the story of how Erin had been diagnosed. It was after Mrs. Wood had described her two trips to the geneticist's office that the moment of insight occurred. For the benefit of the student, I had Mrs. Wood tell us how she and her husband had responded to the news that had been delivered to them by the geneticist.

"At first, we went numb," she replied. "By that point, we both knew there was something wrong with Erin, but we'd prayed it was nothing terrible. To look at Erin back then, you wouldn't think there was anything wrong with her. I mean, she looked and acted pretty much like any other little girl. Yes, her development was slow, but to look at her, you wouldn't think she had something that was going to turn her into the way she is now."

"So first you were numb," I repeated. "Then what happened?"

"Well, of course, once the news sank in, the crying started. The doctor gave us a copy of the results of the tests. He also gave us a booklet called 'Your Child with Sanfilippo Syndrome.' I spent the next few days looking at the results, looking at that booklet, and bursting into tears. My husband went to work—he couldn't stay home—but I could do nothing else. I couldn't care for my children, I couldn't clean the house, I couldn't cook dinner. I was just a basket case."

"How did Erin react?" the medical student asked. I could see the story had sucked her in, and I was happy she was getting something out of this visit.

Mrs. Wood's face broke into a smile. "That's a nice story," she said dreamily toward the medical student. "Like I said, although to look at her now, you may not believe it, back then, Erin looked and acted pretty much like an average four-year-old. She didn't know exactly what was going on, but she saw me crying and was aware that something was wrong. So about three or four days after we'd been to the geneticist the second time, I was sitting on a chair in the living room, soaking yet another Kleenex, and she came to me with one of her old baby bottles filled with milk. Now, Erin had stopped using a bottle when she was two. I don't know where she'd found that bottle or how she'd managed to get the milk into it, but somehow she had. She handed it to me and said, 'Here, Mommy. For you.' 'What's this for?' I asked her. 'You crying, Mommy,' she replied, and in her own way, using the few words she had, she let me know that when she'd been little and cried, I always gave her a bottle of milk and that made her feel better. Because I was crying, she figured that giving me a bottle would make me feel better.

"Of course, her giving me the bottle only made me cry more. I hugged that little girl and cried and we stayed like that for what seemed like hours. When I finally let her go, Erin just turned and walked out of the living room and it was over. That was the only reaction we ever got from her."

The office was silent for a while after Mrs. Wood finished telling us that story. I don't know about the medical student, but fighting off tears, I was too choked up to talk. I had only known Erin more or less in the state in which she exists today. Before hearing her mother's story, I could never even imagine her any other way. Hearing that story was like having a lightbulb switched on in the room. Finally, I understood why Mrs. Wood continued to take such exquisite care of Erin, why the family put up with so many disruptions, why the Woods would never even consider placing the child in a chronic care facility. It was not because of the being Erin was now: it was because of the girl Erin had been back then, before I knew her.

I came to know Erin and her family after the ripples that had been created by her diagnosis had dissipated. Not having lived through the initial disturbance, not having been involved in the family's care back when Erin's condition had first been diagnosed, I could never have comprehended what was motivating their actions in the present. The story of that sweet little girl trying to comfort her grieving mother was all the information I needed.

ERIN LIVED TO be 22, older than most children with Sanfilippo syndrome, her longevity undoubtedly a consequence of the superb treatment provided by her parents in the latter years of her life. By the time she died, I had published an essay about her in the *American Journal of Medical Genetics.* Her parents were so proud of it, so happy that their daughter's life had been commemorated, that they exhibited a framed copy of the essay at Erin's funeral for everyone in attendance to read.

Held in the chapel of a funeral home near Erin's house in Connecticut, the place was standing room only. In addition to family and friends, attendees included all the doctors who had cared for Erin during her life, her home attendants and teachers, her physical and occupational therapists. Sitting in the chapel, I was amazed by how this young woman who could not communicate had touched the lives of so many people.

Although the funeral should have been a time for peace and solace, there was a lot of tension in the air. This was caused by developments that had recently taken place in the lives of Erin's parents. To explain the cause of the tension, I need to go back to events that occurred a year before Erin's death.

At the medical school at which I work, it's become tradition that the final session of Molecular and Cellular Foundations in Medicine, a required course for first-year students, is turned over to me to present patients to the class. The goal is to show the students that there's a human basis to the complex molecular and biochemical concepts they've learned about over the past few months. The year Erin was 21, I asked her parents if they would bring Erin and speak to the class. I thought the students, who had learned about the mucopolysaccharidoses, would get something out of meeting Erin and hearing the story of her diagnosis.

Families respond differently to my invitation to speak to the medical students. Some turn me down cold, offering no explanation (although I know better than to ask, I'm pretty sure A.C. Sheridan's mom, who demands so much privacy, would have fallen into this group); others, after considering the request for a while, ultimately turn down the invitation, saying they'd rather not bare their souls and air personal laundry in front of 180 strangers; but still others, either immediately or after thinking about it, do choose to accept, gravitating naturally toward using their life's experience to play the role of educator. Mr. and Mrs. Wood accepted without hesitation.

The session, which was scheduled to last for 60 minutes, had been going very well. Sitting at the front of the large lecture hall that seated more than 200 students, were, from left to right, Mr. Wood, Erin, Mrs. Wood, and me. Through the entire event, Erin sat in her wheelchair, her heavy head resting on her chest. As usual, she made no sound. My role was to get the Woods to tell their story. Though clearly nervous, they were able to get through the entire tale, with Mrs. Wood doing most of the talking. The students were clearly touched by Mrs. Wood's story about Erin and the baby bottle filled with milk. Looking around the room, I noticed that most of the students had tears in their eyes.

And then it happened. The hour was almost over. To tie things up, I realized that I had to get them to talk about their daughter's death, an event that was inevitable and undoubtedly not that far off. The couple had devoted their recent lives to caring for their daughter, sacrificing everything, their time, their money, their own comfort, so that Erin could live at home; her death was clearly going to change things. So, somewhat naively, I asked this question: "Have you thought of what your lives will be like after Erin's gone?"

I don't know exactly what caused him to say it. Maybe he decided that this was finally his opportunity to say what had been on his mind for a long time; perhaps no one had asked him the question before. But without hesitation, as if by some reflex, Mr. Wood replied, "When Erin dies, our marriage will be over. My wife and I have nothing in common anymore except Erin. Once she's gone, we'll have nothing holding us together. I assume we'll get a divorce."

As my mouth dropped open, I could hear a collective gasp coming from 180 throats. Looking over, I saw that Mrs. Wood's mouth had dropped open as well; it was clear that the couple had never discussed this before, had never even talked about Erin's death, let alone made plans for the time after she was gone. (This was not all that surprising; although some families, like the Thompsons, feel comfortable planning out every detail of their child's funeral and their future lives, others find themselves unwilling or unable to discuss among themselves anything that might happen after that day.) I was too tongue-tied to say anything other than, "Does anyone have any questions?" No one was able to say a word. And that's how the session ended.

After this session, when they'd had a chance to talk the whole thing over, Mr. Wood had vowed to his wife that he would not leave until Erin was gone. However, he actually lasted at home for only about nine more months. One morning after he'd left for work, Mrs. Wood received a letter hand-delivered by a messenger from her husband that said he had taken a job in Rochester, New York, and would not be returning to the house. Mrs. Wood tried to hold it together for Erin's sake, but her depression was taking over. And then the final event: one morning about six weeks after her husband left home, Mrs. Wood found Erin dead in her bed.

The funeral was the first time that the parents had seen each other since Mr. Wood had sent the letter. Needless to say, things were extremely awkward, and this was reflected in the funeral itself, which was the shortest one I've ever been to, lasting no more than ten minutes.

Mrs. Wood has since managed to put her life back together. After a long period of depression, after months of trying to find something worthwhile to fill the hours, she went back to work in a doctor's office. "I'm using what Erin taught me," she told me last year during one of our regular phone conversations. "Through my work, Erin's spirit lives on."

CHAPTER 11

No Sweat!

T HE MOMENT I saw Daryn Jordan, I got a queasy feeling in my stomach. From experience, I knew this wasn't a good sign: I usually get this sensation only when I'm standing in the presence of a patient with some terrible, life-threatening, but as yet undiagnosed disease. So, from his appearance, because of the sound of his cry, but mostly because of the presence of that feeling in my gut, I knew Daryn was in trouble.

I'd been asked to see Daryn by Dr. Albert Reynolds, a very senior pediatric neurologist who'd admitted the seven-month-old to the Children's Hospital's infants' unit for an evaluation.

"I'm worried about this child," Dr. Reynolds told me on the phone. "According to his parents and his pediatrician, less than a month ago, he was doing everything a six-month-old should be doing: he was smiling, rolling over, sitting without support, babbling, everything. But over the past few weeks, he's lost all of this. When I saw him yesterday, he was listless, cranky, and floppy as a dishrag. He can't sit even when propped up, and the only sound he makes is this high-pitched cry."

"He's regressing," I said.

"It sure seems like it," Dr. Reynolds replied. "I admitted him this morning for a workup. We've got him scheduled for an EEG, an MRI, a spinal tap, a metabolic screen, and a battery of blood tests. I've asked ophthalmology to see him, and I'd also like you to evaluate him, to see if you can figure out some genetic explanation for his problems."

When I told him I'd get to the floor as soon as I could, Dr. Reynolds asked if I'd expedite the consult: "This has to be done fast," he explained. "Since the Fourth of July weekend starts tomorrow, we've got to get everything done today or he'll wind up stuck here waiting for the next four days."

I promised I'd go immediately and, after hanging up the phone, I began the trek up to the hospital's inpatient wing.

Up on the infants' floor, I found Daryn in a semiprivate room. He was alone there, lying flat on his back in a hospital crib, and as I've already mentioned, he didn't look great. His limbs were outstretched and flaccid. He cried constantly in the high-pitched whine Dr. Reynolds had described, the kind of cry I knew pointed to the fact that something was very wrong with his brain. That's when I felt that queasiness, the blip from my gastrointestinal radar that told me that Al Reynolds's impression had been correct: I was almost certain the kid had a neurodegenerative disease.

A closer exam only reinforced my feeling. Daryn's posture and cry weren't the only features that were concerning: with a pallid complexion, dark circles under his eyes, and a wasted-appearing body, he looked chronically ill. And his head seemed too large for that wasted body, a feature that suggested that something, possibly an abnormal chemical, was building up to toxic levels in his neurons. Closing my eyes, thinking through the evidence, I silently prayed that I was wrong, that this baby might not have a neurodegenerative disease. But I knew he did; I was sure he did.

BECAUSE OF THEIR unforgiving courses, the neurodegenerative diseases, a group of rare but devasting syndromes, are among the most dreaded disorders in all of pediatrics. Caused by separate genetic flaws that lead to the deficiency of specific enzymes, these diseases—of which the mucopolysaccharidoses that affected Erin Wood and Tommy Sweeney are one category—are characterized by the buildup in the tissues and blood of toxic chemicals. Though these chemicals are actually normally occurring intermediates in complex biochemical pathways, the lack of the essential enzyme that would normally break them down and allow them to be excreted causes them to build up to high concentrations. The substances are then stored in the liver, spleen, bones, and, most devastating, the brain, where their accumulation leads to impaired functioning and ultimately death.

It's the natural history of these disorders that makes them so devastating: they take seemingly normal, healthy infants and systematically destroy them. Consider Tay-Sachs disease: in the womb, the fetus with Tay-Sachs is fine; although he or she suffers from a complete lack of hexosaminidase A (hex A), an enzyme that breaks down substances called GM_2

gangliosides, no problem occurs because of the presence of adequate amounts of hex A in the mother's bloodstream. It's only after birth, after the umbilical cord has been cut, that these gangliosides begin to accumulate. Gradually building up in the neurons, the chemical insidiously makes its presence known after the first six months have passed, manifesting itself first through a slowdown and arrest in developmental progress, and then through the loss of previously attained milestones. First, the child is no longer able to sit, and then his or her ability to roll over ceases; the child becomes unable to respond to external stimuli, eventually becoming locked into his or her own world. Children with Tay-Sachs typically spend the last few years of their lives in a vegetative state, cut off from the rest of the world, usually dying of pneumonia or inanition (inability to eat, which leads to lack of food and water) before their fifth birthday. And in virtually all of these neurodegenerative conditions, nothing can be done to alter the course.

Tay-Sachs, like most neurodegenerative diseases, is inherited in an autosomal recessive fashion. As previously described, asymptomatic parents of an affected child each bear one non-working copy of the hex A gene and one working copy. The amount of hex A produced by the working gene, about 50 percent of that found in normal individuals, is enough to keep them in good health. In the affected child, however, because he has inherited one copy of the nonworking gene from each parent, virtually no enzyme is produced; a nearly total lack of the hex A leads to the inability to break down the gangliosides, causing the disease.

Because most of these conditions are rare, being a carrier

is also not all that common. Because both parents need to be carriers (and since the chances are small of a carrier randomly finding someone in the population who is also a carrier), these conditions occur more commonly when the parents are related. In taking a family history, this is a feature geneticists always ask about.

Similarly, another characteristic of many of the neurodegenerative diseases is that they tend to occur more commonly in one particular ethnic group. Tay-Sachs, for instance, is seen mainly in children of Ashkenazi Jews, people who can trace their origin to the town of Suwalki in northeastern Poland, the site where the original mutation is believed to have occurred, while a form of Niemann-Pick disease occurs only in Acadians from western Nova Scotia, and aspartylglucosaminuria is particularly common in people from Finland.

Daryn Jordan was not a member of any of these ethnic groups. He was African American, and without talking with his parents, I couldn't be sure where his family originated. But one fact was certain: both the clinical evidence and my trusty old intestinal barometer pointed to the conclusion that Daryn was affected by a neurodegenerative disease. The exact one still needed to be determined. As I stood over him with my eyes closed, thinking through the course of action that needed to be taken, I jumped ahead to the step in the process I dreaded the most: the informing interview, the meeting with Daryn's parents when I would tell them that their son had a slowly but steadily progressive disease that would kill him by the time he was five. And while I thought about this and prayed I'd be wrong, I sighed to myself in anticipation of that horrible session.

I WAS STILL STANDING over the crib with my eyes closed when a heavyset woman appeared at the room's doorway. "What are you doing to my baby?" she asked in a voice that bore more than a hint of a Caribbean accent.

"I'm Dr. Marion. I'm a geneticist, a doctor who specializes in diseases that run in families. Dr. Reynolds asked me to see your son while he was here."

"It's not anything that runs in my family that's causing my boy to be like this," she replied, entering the room and taking a seat on a chair adjacent to the crib. "It's this heat that's bothering him. He don't like the hot weather and this room is pretty hot!"

She was right about that: the Bronx was stuck in a sweltering early-summer heat wave and the hospital's air-conditioning wasn't doing all that much to make things any better. "Has Dr. Reynolds told you anything about what he's worried about?" I asked.

"Oh, he told me all right," the woman replied. "He thinks my baby has some disease that's causing him to store some kind of stuff in his brain and that stuff in his brain is making him act like he's acting. That man's crazy! Who ever heard of a disease like that?"

"He's right," I said, smiling. I liked this woman, which wasn't a good thing; it would make it more difficult when I had to tell her that the baby had a terminal condition. "There are diseases that can do that. They're very rare, and they tend to run in families. Is there anyone in either your family or in Daryn's father's family who might have had anything like this, where a baby did okay for a while and then started to lose ground?" After she shook her head, I began to take a formal family history.

The Jordan family pedigree was voluminous. Although Daryn was the first child born to his 23-year-old mother and 25-year-old father, both parents were members of large families: Ms. Jordan was the youngest of eight brothers and sisters, while her husband was one of ten children. And most of the siblings had gone on to have many children of their own. But, to the mother's knowledge, not one of those children had died during childhood, was mentally retarded, or had anything similar to the problems that seemed to be plaguing Daryn.

Ms. Jordan and Daryn's father had come to New York only two years before, having lived most of their lives in Trinidad. They were born, raised, and had met and married in Moruga, a small town on the southern coast of the island. And although Ms. Jordan adamantly denied the possibility that she and her husband were cousins, she did admit that Moruga was a small, isolated place, and it certainly was possible that, somewhere back in time, there might be some shared blood.

After I finished constructing the pedigree that illustrated the family history, I explained to Ms. Jordan that although I wasn't sure exactly what was wrong with Daryn, there was a good chance that Al Reynolds's impression was correct. "We won't know for sure until we get back the tests that we're doing," I explained. "When everything's back, we'll have your husband and you come in and we'll explain everything. Do you have any questions?"

She was silent for a few seconds. "Doctor, is my baby going to die?" she asked.

I sighed. "I can't be sure, Ms. Jordan. We'll have a much better idea when we get the tests back."

"Is there anything I can do to help him?" her eyes filling with tears.

"No," I replied. "If he has one of these diseases, there's nothing anyone can do to make him better." I hesitated after saying that, listening to her crying. Then, I added, "The only thing you can do is pray that Dr. Reynolds and I are wrong."

She seemed surprised by this advice. "I'll pray then, Doctor. Thank you."

And with that, I pulled a copy of my card out of my pocket, handed it to her, and silently left the room.

WE KNEW QUICKLY that making a diagnosis in Daryn's case would not be easy. By the time he was discharged late that afternoon, we already had the results of his spinal tap, EEG, MRI, and ophthalmologic exam: all were perfectly normal. Our ability to make a definitive diagnosis therefore depended on the results of the large number of blood tests that had been sent off to obscure labs spread across the United States, results that would take weeks, perhaps months, to come back. We agreed that Dr. Reynolds would act as the quarterback in Daryn's follow-up care, getting the results and scheduling a joint meeting when the abnormal test finally came back.

Months passed. The hot summer of that year turned into a much milder autumn, and I'd heard nothing from Dr. Reynolds about Daryn or his test results. I'd almost forgotten the child completely when, in early November, I got a call from the boy's mother. "Dr. Marion, I'm calling to tell you that your advice worked."

"What advice?" I asked.

"You told me to pray, remember? You told me to pray you and Dr. Reynolds were wrong, and I prayed, and now Daryn is better. My boy is fine. He is sitting up again. He is talking again. And now he is starting to stand. You and Dr. Reynolds were wrong. It is a miracle!"

"That's very nice," I replied, not believing a word the woman was saying. I wasn't surprised by what I was hearing: denial is an almost universal stage in the mourning process through which Ms. Jordan had to pass before she finally could come to accept her son's diagnosis. I had no doubt she was in denial; once they begin to lose milestones, kids with neurodegenerative diseases never regain them, and they certainly never reach new ones.

Realizing that her denial would only be temporary and that sooner or later she'd need our support, I asked her to bring Daryn to see me for a follow-up visit the next week. After hanging up, I called Dr. Reynolds. "I just got off the phone with Daryn Jordan's mother," I told him. "Have you seen Daryn recently?"

"No," the neurologist replied, "not since he left the hospital. There's really been no need to: all the tests came back normal. I don't have anything to tell her."

"So you don't know how he's doing?"

"Not at all. I assume by this point he's probably close to vegetative."

"His mom just told me he's making progress. She says he's starting to stand holding on."

"Sure he is," Dr. Reynolds responded. "And tomorrow, I'll be retiring to the villa I'm planning to buy in the South of France. Sounds like heavy denial. I wish I knew what was wrong; at least then we'd be able to give her a realistic picture of the future. Unfortunately, it looks like this is going to be one of those cases where the diagnosis isn't made until we get a look at his brain on the autopsy table."

"Well, I'm going to see him in my office next week, just to keep track of him," I responded. "I'll let you know what I find."

"Absolutely. And please let me know if there's anything I can do to help," he replied before we hung up.

ALL MS. JORDAN'S praying must have helped, because as she'd told me on the phone, Dr. Reynolds and I had been dead wrong about Daryn Jordan. It turned out that Ms. Jordan wasn't in heavy denial, and she wasn't lying about her son's progress. When they came to my office the following Wednesday, I was amazed to find that Daryl *was* sitting up by himself; he *was* standing. I stared at him as he stood smiling at me, holding tightly onto his mother's knee, while she told me the story: "For the first few months he was weak, the way you saw him in the hospital that time. Every morning I went to church and asked God to make my baby healthy. My husband, he say to me, 'Why you waste your time? This boy is never going to be any good.' But I kept on, every day. And then, all of the suddenly, it started to work. One morning, my son smiled at me; the next week, he was rolling over. Then he started to crawl. After that, he was sitting up again. That's when I called you. He doesn't have that bad disease Dr. Reynolds said he had anymore, does he? He's cured of that, isn't he?"

I had to admit that Daryn certainly was not now acting like a child with a neurodegenerative disease. But what was it that was wrong with him? Although bigger, stronger, and more alert than the child I'd seen five months before, Daryn still didn't look right: still appearing chronically ill, his skin retained the sallow appearance; it was wrinkled and puckered, especially around his eyes, and the dark circles were still present. But there were some other things about Daryn that were troubling, features that, although they'd been present when he'd been seven months old, hadn't made much of an impression. They were catching my attention now, though.

The boy was bald. His too-large-for-his-body head bore only a few strands of coarse silver hair. And he was edentulous: there was not a single tooth in either his upper or lower jaw. Though not that striking in a seven-month-old, his complete lack of hair and teeth certainly raised an eyebrow in a one-year-old.

It was at that moment that the pieces of the puzzle finally clicked into place.

Excitedly, I began to question Ms. Jordan about the boy's post-hospitalization course: "When exactly did he start to smile at you again?"

She thought for a few seconds. "The end of September," she finally said.

I nodded. "And he started to roll over and crawl in early October?"

This time she nodded.

"And he sat toward the end of October?"

"That's right," she said. "And he started to stand last week. He's cured, right, Dr. Marion? The praying cured him."

"Not exactly cured," I replied, going on with the questions. "I notice he doesn't have any teeth and doesn't have a lot of hair. Did he ever have any teeth or more hair?"

She laughed. "Dr. Marion, you think I shaved my baby's head? You think I pulled out his teeth? No, this is the way God made him, the way he always has been."

"During the summer, did you notice if he ever perspired?"

"Per . . . what?"

"Perspired. You know, did he ever sweat?"

"Oh, sweat. No, Daryn never sweats. Even on the hottest day, he stayed dry as a bone. Is that bad?"

"Not bad," I replied. "It's just Daryn. Ms. Jordan, do you sweat?"

"No. I'm like Daryn. I'm dry like a bone, too. And I don't like the heat: I couldn't stand summers in Trinidad. That's why we came to New York; I made my husband move. I was always too hot in my home. Still can't stand summer, but it's not as bad here as it was back home."

"Does your hair grow fast?"

"Grow fast?" she repeated with a laugh, running her hand through her short, wiry hair. "Dr. Marion, my hair doesn't grow at all. I haven't cut it in more than a year."

"Do you have any trouble with your teeth?"

She thought about it for a few seconds. "No trouble. I still have some baby teeth, though. They never fell out. Is that bad?"

"Not bad," I replied. "It's just you. You and Daryn. Ms. Jordan, I know what's wrong with your son. He doesn't have a disease like the one Dr. Reynolds and I thought. He has a condition called hypohidrotic ectodermal dysplasia."

"Hypo . . . what?"

"Hypohidrotic ectodermal dysplasia. It's a condition that causes problems with structures that come from cells in the body that are called the ectoderm. What it means is that Daryn's body has trouble making teeth and hair. It means that all his life, Daryn will have thin hair that will grow slowly and he'll always be missing most of his teeth."

The mother looked shocked.

"People with this condition also don't have sweat glands," I continued. "Those are the holes in the skin through which you sweat. Because he doesn't have sweat glands, Daryn doesn't have the ability to sweat."

The mother's look of shock now turned into one of puzzlement. "No sweat glands? That's crazy. I never heard of such a thing."

"No, it's true," I told her, reaching for my copy of the book *Smith's Recognizable Patterns of Human Malformations* and opening it to the section on hypohidrotic ectodermal dysplasia. "See?"

"These pictures do look a little like Daryn," she said after studying the photos. "But where did my son get this? Did he catch it from someone?"

"I wouldn't exactly say he caught it," I replied. "It's inherited in what's called an X-linked recessive pattern, which means it's passed down from mothers who have mild symptoms to their sons, who are more severely affected. That's why I asked you about your hair and your teeth and your sweating. You have a mild case of it, but Daryn's condition is much worse."

She considered this for a few seconds. "Well, my son does look like these pictures, and he sure doesn't have any hair or teeth. Maybe he does have this. But so what? Daryn had a brain problem last summer, not a hair or teeth or sweat-gland problem. What does this have to do with what was wrong with him?"

"Ms. Jordan, this is what caused all of Daryn's problems. Don't you see? Sweat is the body's way of cooling itself off when it gets overheated. If you don't have sweat glands, your temperature keeps going up, and eventually you just can't function anymore. When was it that you first noticed Daryn was losing his ability to sit up?"

"In the middle of June," his mother answered.

"Just when it got really hot last summer. And he got better in September—"

"When it got cool," the mother interrupted, finally understanding the point.

"Right. Daryn's brain never degenerated. Because he can't sweat, his body couldn't function in the heat. He wilted like a flower that was out of water too long, and he didn't come back to life until the weather cooled off."

AND LIKE A FLOWER, Daryn Jordan blossomed through the next few years. Within a month of that visit to my office, he began walking; by two, he was speaking in sentences; and at five, he entered kindergarten, developmentally and emotionally appropriate for his age. (I did make sure that his classroom was air-conditioned.)

Unquestionably, life has never been easy for Daryn: he's continued to have problems with the heat during summer. But both he and his mother found ways of coping. They learned to carry a spray bottle of ice water wherever they went, from which Ms. Jordan would spritz both her son's forehead and her own whenever life got a little too hot. On the worst days, she found that taking him to the supermarket and letting him play in the frozen food section almost always perked him up.

We take so much for granted. Though we understand the consequences of our heart failing to beat and of our lungs failing to suck in and blow out air, and we recognize the difficulties presented by failure of our senses to do their job, we rarely give any thought to the importance of more mundane functions. Who considers what effect not being able to feel pain would be like? When do we give a second thought to our ability to stand from a sitting position without passing out? And when does anyone ever imagine what life would be like if we lacked the ability to sweat?

By his ability to persevere, through his hard work, Daryn Jordan has been able to overcome his unusual disability and now leads a relatively normal life. But it hasn't been easy. No, I can safely say that Daryn Jordan's life has certainly not been a "no sweat" existence.

Postscript

HYPOHIDROTIC ECTODERMAL DYSPLASIA (HED) is an unusual disorder. It's one of a small group of conditions in which all the features are visible immediately upon coming into contact with the affected individual. As with a person affected by albinism (technically called oculocutaneous albinism, because it involves both the skin and the eyes), you can tell that someone has HED from across a room, because the boy or man has no hair and no teeth. The obviousness of the diagnosis, the fact that everyone can recognize that there's something different about this person, has profound effects on the individual's social development. When I wrote this essay, Daryn had been doing extremely well. Today, as a teenager, he has serious psychological problems: he has few friends, has never had a girlfriend or found a girl who is interested in being with him, and he spends most of his time alone in his room. He is clearly depressed; although I tell him at every visit that it's what's inside that really counts, and have repeatedly referred him for counseling, he's resisted reaching out for help. Experience tells me that he'll be better when he hits his twenties, but that doesn't make it any easier on any of us who know him and care for him today.

Like many diagnoses of genetic disorders, Daryn's was made on the basis of his clinical findings. At that time, although it was clearly known that the condition was an X-linked recessive disorder, the actual genetic basis responsible for HED had not yet been identified. In 1996, Juha Kere and colleagues at the University of Helsinki in Finland found that a gene called *EDA* was disrupted in patients with HED who had a translocation involving the X chromosome.[1] This is an unbelievable opportunity, an experiment of nature, a chance break in a chromosome found in a child with a genetic disorder that points us to the exact spot in the genome where the responsible gene resides. Quickly, in studying other children with HED, this group identified mutations in this gene, changes (rather than breaks) in the DNA pattern that also led to these symptoms.

This work also led to the development of an animal model of HED and at least a cursory understanding of what the protein produced by the gene does. We now know that *EDA* produces a protein called ectodysplasin A, which is a member of a class of proteins known as the tumor necrosis factor-related ligand family, and that it plays a role in early interaction between epithelial and mesenchyme cells, embryonic forerunners of the skin and its derivatives. Not surprisingly, the protein is expressed in hair follicles, sweat glands, and cells that give rise to the teeth. Although these facts are known, the reason that a change in the gene (which leads to abnormal ectoplasmin-A protein) causes the features we see in affected individuals is still not understood.

This is not unusual in clinical genetics. Even with all the advances that have been made in our understanding of how genes work, even though the genome has been sequenced, we geneticists still make diagnoses based on the clinical features present in our patients, and we treat the problems that arise as a result of these clinical features. DNA testing for mutations in *EDA* is important, but it's important to confirm our clinical impression, and for purposes of providing genetic counseling to the family; it is rarely helpful in treating the patient. As has been the case for its entire history, most of the practice of medical genetics comes down to the clinician sitting in the clinic with the family, listening to the history, performing the physical exam, and trying to put the pieces of the puzzle together.

CHAPTER 12

The Skeleton in
Mr. Anderson's Closet

I N MY WORK, I get to rummage around in places where other health care professionals never get to go. Because the family history is such an important part of my job, because the finding of even subtle symptoms and signs in siblings, parents, and grandparents is so essential in determining whether a condition has been passed from one generation to the next, we geneticists spend a lot of our time delving into the past, searching for the proverbial skeletons that may be hidden away in a family's closet. Often the skeletons lie buried under layers of denial, shame, disappointment, and pain; sometimes, however, they are right at the surface, obvious, impossible to miss even with the naked eye. The latter was true of Carl Anderson's skeleton.

One morning about five years ago, I was called to the nursery at University Hospital to see a baby who'd been born the night before. Over the phone Amanda Stern, the resident who'd been on call, told me that as soon as she saw the kid, she knew something was wrong. "Her vital signs were fine, and her color and muscle tone were normal," Amanda explained, "but there's something really weird about her. She has the longest fingers and toes I've ever seen on a baby. She looks like a spider. I've never seen a baby with Marfan syndrome, but if I had to guess, I'd say this one's got it."

Standing over the child a few minutes later, I quickly came to the same conclusion. At 25 inches from the top of her head to the bottom of her heel, this infant, officially known to the nursery staff as "Baby Girl Anderson," was longer than any other newborn I'd ever seen. And it wasn't just her length that made her appearance so striking: her body was all out of proportion. Although she seemed to have a normal-sized trunk and head, her arms and legs were extremely long and thin; and, as Amanda had said, her fingers and toes were amazing, appearing as if they were the extremities of a spider. I had to agree with Amanda's impression: although she was only a few hours old and I knew nothing about her family history, I was willing to bet that this baby had Marfan syndrome.

AS IN THE CASE of Baby Girl Anderson, it was the appearance of his patient's limbs that in 1896 first struck Antoine Marfan, a French pediatrician, and caused him to describe the syndrome that now bears his name.[1] Like Gabrielle, Dr. Marfan's five-year-old patient, people affected with the disorder have a wide spectrum of unusual skeletal findings. Their unusual height is the result of disproportionate elongation of their legs. As a result of laxity of their ligaments, affected individuals are loose-jointed and have flat feet. Also, their chests frequently either have a caved-in appearance (a condition known as pectus excavatum) or bulge outward (pectus carinatum). They have scoliosis (curvature of the spine), and they tend to be skinny; affected individuals complain that they have trouble bulking up and building muscle. Although they may drink high-calorie supplements and work out many hours every day, they tend to remain thin and relatively weak.

But in the century since Dr. Marfan's original description, it's become clear that the disorder, which occurs in 1 in every 10,000 live births, consists of a lot more than just these unusual skeletal findings. Because the underlying abnormality involves a defect in the formation of connective tissue, the glue that holds the body together, other major organ systems are affected, systems that, because of the anomalies that characteristically occur, significantly interfere with the affected person's quality of life and, more important, if untreated, frequently lead to an early death.

The eyes of patients with Marfan syndrome are abnormal. Affected individuals tend to be exceptionally nearsighted, their myopia so severe that degeneration of the vitreous and retina may occur, leading to worsening of their vision. Also, like the ligaments that function in the skeletal system, the suspensory ligament, the structure that holds the lens of the eye in place, is less firm than it should be; weakness in the suspensory ligament leads to ectopia lentis, dislocation of the lens. The net effect of all this is that, with the passage of time, patients with Marfan syndrome often develop severe and disabling visual impairment.

But the impairment caused by their visual disturbances is a relatively minor complaint compared with what happens in the cardiovascular system. Because of the generalized flaw in the connective tissue that is the underlying problem in the disorder, the walls of the aorta, the large artery that carries blood away from the heart to the remainder of the body, is weakened. Over the course of time, as blood spurts at high pressure out of the heart into the aorta, the wall's weakness leads to a progressive thinning of that wall and dilatation of the aorta, known as an aneurysm. Eventually, usually when the artery has dilated so much that the diameter is more than twice its normal size, the aorta actually tears apart; the aneurysm dissects, flooding the chest with blood and rapidly resulting in death (as it did in the cases of Flo Hyman, a member of the U.S. Olympic women's volleyball team in 1988; the playwright Jonathan Larson, who died the night of the final dress rehearsal of his musical, *Rent,* in 1996; and the actor John Ritter, who died suddenly in 2003).

Without treatment, most individuals with Marfan syndrome reach that terrible point at which their weakened aorta bursts, in their forties or fifties. But early death due to dissection of an aortic aneurysm is not the only bad news in this condition; because it's inherited in an autosomal dominant manner, passed along from affected parent to affected child, each offspring of an affected individual has a 50 percent chance of also being affected. Since in the majority of cases, prenatal diagnosis is not possible, affected parents must either decide to take a chance and hope that their child is not affected or (if they're not the gambling type) decide not to have children at all.

WHEN I FINISHED examining Baby Girl Anderson, I went to talk with Amanda. After telling the resident that I agreed with her impression and complimenting her on her clinical acumen, I asked if she knew anything about the child's parents. Amanda told me that although the baby's mother, Mrs. Anderson, was blind for reasons that hadn't been spelled out in the prenatal chart, she was just barely over five feet tall and appeared to have none of the skeletal manifestations of Marfan syndrome. Curious about the mother's ophthalmologic condition, I immediately went to speak with her.

I found Mrs. Anderson alone and asleep in a bed on the postpartum ward. After a quick look, I found myself once again agreeing with Amanda Stern's assessment: although her eyes looked abnormally small, the result, undoubtedly, of the condition that caused her blindness, Mrs. Anderson otherwise looked completely normal. "If this baby's got Marfan," I thought, "she either inherited it from her father or got it due to a new mutation." While I was thinking about this, the woman began to stir. "Mrs. Anderson?" I asked after seeing her raise her head and look around.

"Who's there?" she asked, turning her head from side to side, trying to pick up some signal about the stranger who had invaded her room.

After introducing myself, shaking her hand, and congratulating her on the birth of her first child, I asked how she was feeling.

"I'm all right," she responded, rapidly, trying to focus on me. "Is there something wrong with my baby?"

"She's absolutely fine right now," I replied, taking a seat

at the woman's bedside. "She's pink and comfortable, and her heart and lungs seem to be working just fine. But she looks a little unusual. She's very long and thin—"

"Is there something wrong with that?" the woman interrupted, more anxious.

"It looks to us like the baby might have a condition called Marfan syndrome. Have you ever heard of it?"

The mother thought for a moment and finally replied, "No. Should I have?"

"It's a problem that sometimes runs in families. It's usually passed from parent to child. People who have it tend to be tall and thin and have problems with their eyes and their hearts. Since we're concerned about Marfan syndrome in the baby, I was just wondering whether you or her father might have it."

"No one ever told me I had it," the woman responded. "I do have problems with my eyes, but that's because I was born with cataracts. That's why I have trouble seeing. But as far as I know, there's nothing else wrong with me. And my husband's never said anything about any syndrome or anything. He is much taller than me, though—"

"How tall?" I interrupted.

"I'm not sure," she answered. "Since I can't see so well, I've never really had a good look at him. It's not something we ever talked about. But he is very tall. And very thin."

"Does he have any other problems with his health?" I asked.

"Well, he has low vision; it's not as bad as mine, though. He can at least get around by himself. I've been blind since birth; he only started to lose his vision when he was a teenager. I'm not exactly sure what happened to him."

With the additional evidence of tall stature and eye disease, I was now just about certain that Baby Girl Anderson's father had Marfan syndrome. But why wouldn't his wife know about his condition? Was it possible that the diagnosis had never been made? "Did anyone suggest that you get genetic counseling during the pregnancy?" I asked.

"I did get genetic counseling!" the new mother replied. "When I was three months pregnant, my midwife sent me to speak to someone in Manhattan about whether my baby might be born with the same eye problem I had. They did some blood tests and told me they couldn't find anything wrong except that I'd been born with cataracts. They said they didn't think my baby would have any problem with her eyes, but they couldn't be a hundred percent sure because they didn't know what was wrong with my husband's eyes. They told me whatever he's got might be genetic."

"Oh, he didn't go with you to talk to the geneticist?" I asked.

"No," she replied, smiling. "He refused. He doesn't like doctors very much."

Just then, in the time it took me to formulate my next question—while I was trying to comprehend how, during the latter part of the 20th century, a man living in New York City who clearly must have had Marfan syndrome could have made it into adulthood without ever having had the diagnosis made—Carl Anderson slipped into the room. At least six and a half feet tall, painfully thin, with enormously long arms and legs and spidery fingers, he looked like a photograph out of a textbook of clinical genetics. After greeting his wife, he kissed her on the cheek, and, trying his best to ignore me, took a seat in a chair by the bedside.

Upon seeing Mr. Anderson, I fell silent.

Mrs. Anderson began to fill him in about what I was doing in the room: "This is one of the doctors who are taking care of the baby. They're worried she might have some problem. Something called Murphy's syndrome?"

"Marfan syndrome," Mr. Anderson corrected, still ignoring me. "And they're right. She does have it. I have it, too."

This statement apparently shocked Mrs. Anderson, but it put me back on track. "How is your health?" I asked Mr. Anderson.

"I'm okay," he replied. "I have my good days and my bad days."

"Where have you been going for your medical care?"

"I used to see some doctors at Manhattan Hospital," he responded, "but I stopped going there a long time ago. They weren't doing anything for me. Every time I went for an appointment, all they ever did was stare at me like I was some kind of a circus freak or something, and tell me I was going to die when I was 45. Who needs that? I know how I look, and I don't need someone to tell me how much longer I have to live."

"Why didn't you tell me you had this thing?" Mrs. Anderson asked, obviously startled by her husband's disclosure.

"Right, and what would you have done? I tell you I've got Marfan syndrome and I'm going to die in 20 years, and the first thing you'd do is take off. And you know that more than anything else in life I wanted to have a kid. If you found out that this disease was inherited and that there was a 50-50 chance that any kid I had would get it, you'd never have gotten pregnant. By not telling you, at least now we have this baby."

During the minutes that followed, Mrs. Anderson tried to explain to her husband that she loved him deeply, regardless of whether he had Marfan syndrome or any other disorder, and that she would be happy to have a baby who was like him. I told him about the breakthroughs that had occurred in the management of the cardiac and vascular complications of the disease—advances that, with the combination of medication, close medical follow-up, and surgical replacement of the weakened aorta with a graft before it reached the point at which it was ready to rupture, would almost guarantee that Mr. Anderson would survive into his sixties or seventies.

That afternoon, echocardiograms (sonographic tests looking at the structures of the heart) were performed on both father and daughter, who had been named Valerie. Thankfully, although both had evidence of widening of their aortic roots, neither's aortic diameter was yet in the danger zone, the region at which we'd have to act. Valerie left the hospital after an uncomplicated two-day stay in the nursery. With frequent follow-up appointments, she and her father have done exceedingly well; to this point, neither has required surgical intervention. And last year, Mrs. Anderson gave birth to the couple's second child, another girl, this one named Katherine. Unlike her sister and father, Katherine is unaffected with Marfan syndrome.

SINCE VALERIE'S BIRTH, I've gotten to know Carl Anderson fairly well. An intelligent, sensitive man, he reads a great deal (in spite of his low vision) and keeps up with developments in research being conducted on the disease that affects him and his daughter. During one of his recent visits, we even got into a heated discussion about whether Abraham Lincoln might have had Marfan syndrome. Carl strongly believes that the 16th president of the United States was affected with what he calls "my disease." I'm not convinced. I wrote about Lincoln's physical findings and why I believe he did not have Marfan syndrome in a book called *Was George Washington Really the Father of our Country? A Clinical Geneticist Looks at World History* (Boston: Addison-Wesley, 1994).

But of all the discussions we've had, the most poignant have involved what having Marfan syndrome has meant to Carl Anderson.

"As far back as I can remember," he told me during one of the family's regular checkups a couple of years ago, "even before they told me I had this thing, I knew I was different. When I was real little, four or five, the kids around our neighborhood used to call me names all the time, like spider boy, freak face, or scarecrow. It always tore me apart inside. I didn't know what to do, so I'd just start crying and run home to my mother. Neither of my parents had Marfan syndrome, so they had no idea how to handle me. My mother would just tell me to stay home and find something to do around the house. She thought hiding was the answer to my problems.

"But once I started school, it got harder for me to hide at home. That's when things really got tough. I used to get into fights nearly every day. A kid would call me 'freak' or 'ugly,' and I'd be on him in a second. Only problem was, I was so weak, I'd always get the crap beat out of me. Nobody would stand up for me; I never had any friends. Anytime I showed interest in a girl, she'd just make fun of me. By the time I was in fourth grade, I'd had it. I never wanted to go to school anymore. I'd wake up in the morning and complain to my mother that I was feeling sick, hoping she'd let me stay home. Lots of times I'd whine so much, she'd give in to me. I'd stay home in bed, crying to myself. I was always depressed. And the people at school never gave a damn about whether I showed up or not. My teachers and the principals, they all thought of me as a troublemaker, so they were happy to have me out of there. I'm not dumb, but I was always a rotten student. I just never made it to school enough days in a row to learn anything."

The cumulative effects of having an inherited disease touched every aspect of Carl Anderson's life. It was his Marfan syndrome that had caused him to develop cataracts at age 16, a complication that ultimately led to the loss of most of his vision, thus severely limiting his career opportunities and his ability to work. (He currently works as a clerk at a candy stand in one of New York City's branch post offices, a job given to him by a city agency that provides services to individuals with low vision.) It was his Marfan syndrome that, because of the predicted early demise that accompanies the illness, had caused him to adopt such a fatalistic attitude toward life. It was the Marfan syndrome that had caused him to appear different—to look, in his words, like a freak—in the eyes of those who populated the world around him. It had been the skeletal manifestations that had caused him to become the brunt of endless teasing from his peers, the Marfan-induced body habitus (i.e., physique) that had led to his lifelong episodes of depression and the nearly daily fights of his childhood, fights that were inevitably lost because of the weakness of his muscles, another contribution of the syndrome. And it had been his unusual morphology and the toll taken by all of these other contributing factors that had led Carl Anderson to develop such a poor self-image. He had even chosen a wife who was literally blind to his faults, and he was terrified to admit to her that he was afflicted with a disorder for fear that she would immediately abandon him, that she would refuse to bear his children, that she would choose to abort a fetus rather than risk having it born similarly affected. Although intelligent and sensitive, Carl Anderson was the man he was largely because of society's reaction to the effects caused by the gene for Marfan syndrome that he carried in every cell in his body.

As a clinical geneticist, there's a price I have to pay for the privilege of rooting around in my patients' pasts. Once I've unearthed a secret, I'm obligated to help the individual and his or her family deal with the consequences. Having unearthed the long, thin skeleton in Carl Anderson's closet, it was part of my job to help him come to grips with who he was. It's not easy to undo the psychological harm caused by a lifetime of taunting and disease, but Carl is clearly making progress.

Postscript

IT TURNED OUT THAT the Manhattan geneticist who told Ms. Anderson that she was not at risk for having children with cataracts was wrong: although Katherine, the second child born to the Andersons, had been unaffected with any genetic disorder, their third child, Ryan, was born with both Marfan syndrome and congenital cataracts. Like Carl's Marfan syndrome, Mrs. Anderson's ophthalmologic condition turned out to also be an autosomal dominantly inherited trait, a fact that was hammered home by the fact that although the couple's fourth child, Eden, was free of Marfan syndrome, she was also born with cataracts. So, in perfect genetic symmetry, of the couple's four children, one inherited both Mr. Anderson's Marfan syndrome and Mrs. Anderson's cataracts, one inherited only Marfan syndrome, one inherited only cataracts, and one inherited neither condition.

These things happen!

As one big happy family, the Andersons come to see me for follow-up visits once a year. I find it amazing to see how, despite what would seem like debilitating disabilities, the children are all well adjusted, polite, smart, and happy. Each child shows both genuine love and respect for his or her siblings; all are clearly in awe of their parents. Thus far, neither Carl nor either of his affected children has required surgery for the cardiac manifestations of Marfan syndrome. And recently, trials with a new medication appear to offer hope that surgery will no longer be a necessity in these individuals. In 2006, an article in *Science* described the profoundly positive effect that the drug losartan, an angiotensin II type 1 receptor inhibitor, has on preventing aneurysms in a mouse model of Marfan syndrome. When given to such mice, losartan not only prevented the development of aneurysms but actually improved aneurysms that had already developed.[2] With trials in humans currently under way, geneticists hope that using this medication beginning early in life will essentially cure the deadly cardiac manifestations of this condition.

In the years since his daughter Valerie's birth, with these new breakthroughs virtually guaranteeing that he will not die anytime soon, Carl Anderson's fatalistic attitude has softened. His lack of self-esteem continues to be a problem, however: no medication, treatment plan, or surgical procedure—no matter how miraculous it might be—could ever overcome the effect that a lifetime of psychological abuse has had on him.

CHAPTER 13

The Right Place, the Right Time

AFTER INTRODUCING MYSELF and leading her into my office, I asked Mrs. Ludlow if she understood why she and her daughter were coming to see me that day.

"Well, to tell you the truth, Doctor, no," she said, sighing.

An attractive woman in her midthirties, Mrs. Ludlow looked tired.

"The only reason we're here is because the Committee on Special Education at our school said they need a report from you before they complete their evaluation of Nicole."

"Why is she being evaluated by the CSE?" I asked.

"She's failing third grade. Nicole's not stupid; she's a bright kid. She's only doing poorly because she's missed so much school this year. They're trying to figure out what to do with her, whether to give her home tutoring, put her in special ed, or make her repeat the year. So they're doing this big evaluation to find out why she has these attacks. But I'm not sure why exactly I'm here, or what you're supposed to be able to add to this evaluation." While Mrs. Ludlow said these words, Nicole, her nine-year-old daughter, sat stone still on a chair across from her mother, silently staring into space.

"Well, I'm a medical geneticist," I explained. "I take care of children with inherited conditions. Is there any reason that the Committee on Special Ed might think Nicole's condition is inherited?"

"Not that I know of," the woman replied. "And frankly, Doctor, I don't have a lot of hope this visit will really accomplish much."

"What makes you think that?" I asked.

"Well, this isn't exactly our first visit to a doctor's office. So far, Nicole's been seen by more than a dozen different medical specialists. Not one of them has been able to tell us exactly what is wrong with her. So, as you might imagine, I'm not very optimistic that this visit will be any different."

"I'll agree it's not likely that I'll be able to add much," I said, suddenly feeling defensive, "but I guess you're already here and we've got nothing to lose by trying. So if it's all right with you, here's what we'll do: First, I'll ask you some questions about Nicole's history; then I'll examine her. And then, we'll talk about where we go from there. Okay?"

Mrs. Ludlow nodded, not very enthusiastically, and I launched into my standard history-taking mode.

"Let's start at the beginning. How much did Nicole weigh when she was born?" As the words were coming out of my mouth, the child began to make a strange noise, a kind of mewing, not unlike the sound our cat makes when it gets stuck in a closet. The noise came from deep inside the girl's throat, not from her vocal chords exactly, but from somewhere farther down. After finishing my question, I stared at Nicole, trying to figure out what she was trying to say.

"Quiet," Mrs. Ludlow said to Nicole. "Don't make that noise. That's a bad noise."

The girl, still staring off into space, immediately became quiet.

"She's not usually like this," Mrs. Ludlow apologized. "She's usually a nice, sweet kid. She's having one of her attacks today. It's these attacks that are the problem."

I stared at the little girl, trying to get her attention. Superficially, she appeared fine: looking at her from across the room, I could identify no abnormal features. But she was certainly acting bizarrely, incoherently, as if she were in a world of her own. Never did she make eye contact with me; not once did she even look in my direction. "Has anyone suggested that Nicole might have autism?" I asked.

"No," the mother responded. "I can understand why you might think that, seeing her the way she is today. But as I said, Doctor, Nicole's usually not like this. She's usually very outgoing. It's only during her attacks that she acts this way. Have you ever heard of autism coming and going like this?"

I shook my head and thought. To say this girl's problem had grabbed my attention was an understatement. "How often do these attacks occur?" I finally asked.

"A couple times a year. Actually, it's good you're seeing her today, so you can understand what I'm talking about. When she's her usual self and I'm trying to explain to people what's wrong with her, people usually think I'm crazy."

"How long does this last?" I asked, not certain what "this" actually referred to.

"I can't tell you for sure," the mother replied. "I never know how long it'll go on. Sometimes she'll be like this for a day or two. Sometimes it'll last longer. The longest one lasted for nearly four weeks."

"Four weeks?" I asked.

Mrs. Ludlow nodded.

"Is there anything that brings them on?"

This time, the mother shook her head no.

"Anything that makes them go away?"

"Not that I can tell," Mrs. Ludlow replied. "They kind of come and go as they like."

"Are they seizures of some kind?" I asked after pondering her response.

"That's what the neurologists have always thought," she replied. "Over the years, Nicole's been seen by five different neurologists. In fact, we saw a new one just a week ago as part of this CSE evaluation. She's been hospitalized three times at three different hospitals for overnight brain wave tests. She's had two CAT scans, one with contrast and one without; an MRI; and about a hundred different blood tests. Every test that's been done has turned out perfectly fine. Every doctor who's ever seen Nicole has told me there's nothing they can find that's wrong with her. Some of them have even accused me of making the whole thing up, of inventing stories about Nicole acting like this because I was crazy. But you're seeing her for yourself. Tell me: how can I be making this up if she's acting like this?"

I told Mrs. Ludlow that, yes, I was seeing her for myself, and I would certainly be willing to swear in a court of law that she hadn't invented Nicole's illness. "You seem to know a lot about medicine," I commented. "Do you have a medical background?"

"No," she replied. "It's just that since I've been through so much with this kid, I've gotten a whole medical education."

"Has anyone tried to treat these episodes with medication?" I asked next.

"Sure," she responded without hesitation. "Every neurologist has started Nicole on some seizure medication. Just last week, the doctor we saw put her on Tegretol. None of these medicines has done even a little bit of good. In fact, if you ask me, some of them have actually made her worse."

"How old was Nicole when the episodes started?" I asked, still groping in the dark, having absolutely no idea what was wrong with this child.

Mrs. Ludlow became energized as she unfolded her daughter's story, the look of exhaustion lifting from her face. The first attack occurred when Nicole was three. Before that, she'd been in excellent health. But then she'd undergone an operation to reduce a displaced fracture in her elbow suffered during a fall. "She was scared going into the surgery," the mother explained, "acting the way any three-year-old would. But then after the operation, it was as if she just never woke up from the anesthesia. It was terrifying: it was like she'd gone into a coma and nobody could do anything to bring her out. At first they thought she suffered brain damage. That's when they did the first CAT scans; it was completely normal. They gave her all kinds of medications, steroids, antibiotics, but nothing would make Nicole wake up. I was sure she was going to die."

I thought for a minute, trying to understand the relationship between the anesthesia and the onset of the illness. Off in the distance, a bell began to toll softly in my head; I knew that that bell signaled the fact that a connection was trying to get made. Nicole's story was beginning to remind me of something, but I still couldn't figure out what. "How long did she stay like that?" I finally asked.

"Two weeks. For two long weeks I sat at her bedside, holding her hand, talking to her, trying to get her to wake up. The doctors came by every morning and every evening and told me they couldn't find anything wrong with her. Then, as suddenly as it had started, one day Nicole just woke up. She opened her eyes, looked up at me, and said 'Hi Mommy,' and that was it."

While her mother was telling this story, Nicole rose from her chair and walked over to my file cabinet. Placing her face against the cold metal wall of the cabinet, she stood rigidly, almost like a statue.

"Is she all right?" I asked.

The mother shrugged. "I guess," she replied. "She's as all right as she ever gets during one of her attacks."

"So after she came out of that first episode, she was back to her old self?" I went on. "As if nothing had happened?"

"As if nothing had happened," she repeated, "except for one thing: the right side of her face drooped. The neurologist told me she had a facial palsy and that she might have it for the rest of her life. Of course, he was wrong: the doctors have been wrong about everything they've predicted about Nicole. Her facial droopiness lasted for about a week. But since then, it's come back a few times, usually during or right after one of the attacks. And sometimes, it's her left side that's affected. It's weird."

On the top page of the legal pad on my desk, I wrote "COMA AFTER ANESTHESIA" on the first line and "RECURRENT FACIAL PALSIES" on the next. The bell inside my head was ringing a little louder now. "So between that first episode and the one she's having now, how many attacks has Nicole had?"

Mrs. Ludlow sighed and thought. "Oh God, I don't know . . . somewhere between 20 and 25, I guess."

Nicole, still pressing her cheek against the wall of the filing cabinet, began softly to make that weird mewing noise again.

"Other than the coma and the facial palsy, what other problems have occurred during the episodes?"

"Please be quiet, honey," the mother said to the child, whose mewing had gradually grown louder. Again, without moving, without making contact with her mother's gaze, the child responded to Mrs. Ludlow's request.

"Let's see," Mrs. Ludlow continued. "Sometimes, her speech gets slurred, as if she's had a stroke."

I wrote "SLURRING OF SPEECH" on the next line of my pad.

"And insomnia. To me, the insomnia is the worst part of it. She can go four or five days in a row without sleeping. I know that's hard to believe, but it's true. So far during this episode, she's been awake for 72 hours or so. And of course, when Nicole's awake, I have to stay awake with her. I'm afraid if I leave her alone, she might wind up hurting herself. So when she doesn't sleep, I don't sleep either."

I wrote "INSOMNIA" on the next line of the pad, realizing that this was undoubtedly the cause of Mrs. Ludlow's haggard appearance. "Anything else?"

"One other thing: she gets terrible pains all over her body, in her neck, in her chest, in her belly, in her back. One time it was so bad, I thought she was having a heart attack; another time, the pain in her belly was so bad that the doctors in the emergency room wanted to take out her appendix."

As I wrote "UNEXPLAINED PAIN" on the pad, I thought I finally knew what was wrong with Nicole; I needed only one more bit of information. "During these attacks, is there anything unusual about Nicole's urine?"

Mrs. Ludlow answered without hesitation, "You're the first person to ask about that, but now that you mention it, there is something weird about her urine. I've always wondered about it, but I never thought to ask. When she's sick, Nicole's urine gets very dark; it can get so dark that it looks like red wine. Does that mean anything?"

It sure did mean something: the girl's dark urine was the key that unlocked her diagnosis. After hearing Mrs. Ludlow's answer, I was almost positive that Nicole had a disorder called acute intermittent porphyria (AIP).

MUCH AS I hate to admit it, my brilliant flash of diagnostic insight wasn't the result of my being smarter than the dozen other physicians who'd seen Nicole before me. This medical epiphany hadn't struck me and failed to strike them because I'd read more articles or had better clinical acumen or had asked more probing questions. No, I'd arrived at my diagnosis due to nothing more than dumb luck. Events in the weeks prior to the Ludlows' visit had primed me to make a diagnosis of porphyria.

At the time of their visit, I was working on a book about historical figures who were affected with genetic diseases. Just the month before, I'd finished a chapter on George III, king of England at the time of the American Revolution. Although George had enjoyed good health through most of his life, his reign, which lasted from 1760 to 1820, had been punctuated by a series of mysterious illnesses, attacks that lasted from a few days to ten years. George's illness, which has come to be known as the Royal Malady, left the king incapacitated and unable to carry out his duties.

There were a lot of similarities between Nicole Ludlow's condition and the one that caused George III, his country, and the colonies so much grief during his lifetime. In both cases, the attacks came and went without warning; in both cases, the episodes were characterized by unusual symptoms such as nerve palsies, altered levels of consciousness, intractable pain that had no identifiable source, and terrible insomnia; in both cases, the urine excreted during these episodes was described as dark or wine-colored; and in both cases, the illness mystified dozens of physicians. In fact, George's illness defied diagnosis throughout his life. The major difference between George III and Nicole Ludlow, of course, is that George, king of the largest nation on earth, was forced to make decisions during these episodes that affected the lives of millions of people, ultimately leading to the American War of Independence, while Nicole was just a little girl.

It was only in 1966, 150 years after George III's death, that a logical explanation for the Royal Malady was finally proposed. After poring over hundreds of pages of medical bulletins issued by the king's personal physician, Macalpine and Hunter, two British physicians, suggested that the features of King George's illness could all be explained by a diagnosis of porphyria.[1]

The porphyrias, a group of rare inherited disorders in which an enzyme needed for production of the protein heme (an essential component of red blood cells) is missing, have two features in common. First, because their bodies cannot produce adequate quantities of heme, affected individuals suffer from anemia. Second, because of the block in the pathway through which heme is produced, precursors of heme build up to extremely high concentrations in the blood, chemicals that in these concentrations are toxic to the skin, the liver, and the central nervous system.

The form of porphyria that affected George III (the same one I thought was present in Nicole Ludlow) does not cause constant symptoms. Under normal circumstances, the level of enzyme that is produced is more than enough to maintain good health. But during times of illness or emotional stress, or following exposure to certain drugs or chemicals, symptoms can occur. So during their lives, people with these forms of porphyria suffer from episodes of seemingly bizarre illness, characterized by unexplained aches, unusual neurologic and psychiatric disturbances, and the passage of abnormally dark urine that's often described as burgundy in color (an effect caused by the presence of excessive amounts of heme precursor in the urine).

The course of Nicole's illness fit the pattern expected in someone with AIP. Her first attack followed exposure to an anesthetic agent, many of which are known to trigger symptoms in affected individuals. During the subsequent years, she'd been treated with a variety of medications, including the anticonvulsant phenobarbital, another well-known exacerbator. In fact, the attack that was at that moment gripping Nicole, causing her to stand with her cheek pressed against the wall of my file cabinet, now again softly mewing, may well have been brought on by treatment with the drug Tegretol (carbamazepine), which she'd begun to take only the week before.

The more I thought about it, the more convinced I became that Nicole had AIP. Although the condition rarely causes symptoms in children as young as Nicole, the features of her illness overlapped too closely with those of AIP to be a coincidence. To prove the diagnosis, I had to complete two tasks. First, since it's inherited in an autosomal dominant fashion, with the mutated gene usually passing from affected parent to affected child, I had to find out which of Nicole's parents also suffered from the condition. And second, using Nicole's blood and urine, I had to prove that she bore evidence of the biochemical abnormalities that cause the disorder. Without telling Mrs. Ludlow about my suspicion, trying to keep as straight a face as possible, I turned my attention to completing the first of these tasks.

IN RESPONSE TO Mrs. Ludlow's question about whether the color of Nicole's urine meant anything, I gave a noncommittal

"Maybe." As I said this, the girl, ungluing her cheek from the wall of the file cabinet, still mewing quietly to herself, came and tried to sit on her mother's lap.

"No, honey, you go sit in that chair," the mother said. Again without hesitation, the girl obeyed.

Then I moved on: "How was your pregnancy with Nicole?" I asked after watching the girl settle in the chair next to her mother's.

"Awful," Mrs. Ludlow replied without any hesitation. "They had to put me in the hospital twice. The first time, I was in my sixth week. I began having terrible stomach pain. My doctor thought I had an ectopic, and he did an exploratory operation on me to see what was going on."

"Did he find anything wrong?" I asked.

"That was the strange thing: they didn't find anything. Everything was fine. Then about a week later, the pain just went away. Weird."

Although I was nearly bursting, realizing Mrs. Ludlow's unexplained episode of pain most likely represented an attack of porphyria, I continued: "What was the story with the second hospitalization?"

"That happened about a month later. They put me in because I was dehydrated. It was terrible: I couldn't stop vomiting. I spent six weeks with an IV in my arm."

Again, this story was consistent with porphyria. "Have you ever had any episodes like Nicole's?" I asked.

The mother shook her head.

Although Mrs. Ludlow's pregnancy history was suspicious (the stress of pregnancy often triggers episodes of the disorder),

I got the final confirmation I needed to fully convince myself while taking the rest of the family history.

Mrs. Ludlow told me that although her husband and his family were all in excellent health, members of her side of the family had had a series of unexplained health problems. "My mother's okay," she said, "but my father's a mess. People think he's a drunk because he has blackouts, but I know for a fact that he never takes a drink because alcohol has always made him sick to his stomach. And then, his sister, she's 80, she's had seizures all her life."

"Anything besides seizures?" I asked.

She shook her head. "That sister has a daughter who's okay—"

"That would be your first cousin?" I interrupted.

"Yes," she continued. "My cousin's okay, but she has a daughter who's been diagnosed with some rare disease. I'm not sure what it's called—"

"Porphyria?" I interrupted, nearly jumping out of my chair.

Mrs. Ludlow's eyes opened wide. "Yes, that's it. How did you know?"

"Mrs. Ludlow, for the past few minutes, I've been thinking that porphyria would explain all of Nicole's problems. Since it's an inherited condition, I've been waiting for you to tell me that someone else in your family has been diagnosed with it."

She seemed mystified. "But how could my cousin and I both have daughters with porphyria if no one else in the family has it?" she asked dubiously.

"Well, in fact, I don't think Nicole and your cousin's daughter are the only ones who have it. I'm pretty sure those problems you had during your pregnancy were episodes of porphyria. And your father's blackouts and his reaction when he drinks alcohol? Those are both probably caused by porphyria, also."

"What about my cousin?" Mrs. Ludlow asked. "She's never been sick—"

"That's one of the strange things about this disease," I interrupted. "The symptoms can vary widely from one person to the next. Some people are sick all the time; others never have a sick day in their lives. I can't explain it better than that."

Mrs. Ludlow considered this. "If she really does have porphyria, and I'm not saying I believe she does, is there anything we can do to help her?" she finally asked.

"Yes, there are plenty of things. We can't cure it, but knowing that she has it may allow us to do things to prevent her from getting so many attacks." I outlined the management that would be instituted, starting with immediately stopping the Tegretol. I also explained that I'd need to get a sample of blood, urine, and stool from Nicole to confirm the diagnosis. When I'd finished, I asked if she had any more questions.

"Just one," Mrs. Ludlow said. "How come you were able to make this diagnosis when so many other doctors hadn't thought of it?"

I shrugged my shoulders, fighting off the urge to tell her that I was much smarter than any of the other doctors who had evaluated Nicole. But what I really should have said was that physicians are just like everyone else. Our lives are influenced by what goes on around us. If we happen to see a patient who has symptoms of a rare disease that was featured on the previous night's episode of *House,* we're going to strongly consider that condition in the differential diagnosis. Although sometimes we'll be right, at other times we're dead wrong.

IT WAS NOT BECAUSE I'm a brilliant diagnostician or because I'm a sensitive listener that I happened to make the diagnosis of acute intermittent porphyria in Nicole and her mother (a diagnosis that was ultimately confirmed through the demonstration of a deficiency of the enzyme uroporphyrinogen I synthase in the girl's red blood cells). Had I seen this family one year before, I'm sure I would have failed, just like the dozen other specialists who had seen Nicole in the past. No, in the case of Nicole Ludlow, I was able to come up with the correct diagnosis simply through dumb luck: the Ludlows and I had managed to run into each other in exactly the right place at exactly the right time.

Dumb luck is an important factor in the lives of clinical geneticists. Dumb luck and hunches, and a little bit of knowledge of weird rare facts, are pretty much all that keep me in business.

NICOLE LUDLOW IS now 21 years old. Despite the optimism I expressed about our ability to manage her problems on the day I first met her and her mother, her life has been far from easy. Through her teenage years, she suffered multiple episodes of porphyria. As a result, she wound up being hospitalized numerous times at numerous facilities, seeking care from additional dozens of physicians. Her parents went through an ugly divorce, adding to her stress. She became addicted to pain medication, kicked her addiction (her health suffering greatly as a result of the fact that the treatment for her addiction triggered attacks of her condition), only to become addicted again. Even though we all knew her diagnosis, even though we knew the steps that needed to be taken to protect her from her disease, all of this happened because in addition to having porphyria, Nicole was also a fairly typical adolescent and, like most adolescents, she was dead set against doing whatever it was her parents or her doctors wanted her to do. Adolescence can be a tough time for most children and their families, but it can be exceptionally difficult for kids who have a chronic disease.

At the age of 19, Nicole graduated from high school and, with her boyfriend, moved to Atlanta, trying to get as far away from her parents as she could. It was during her time in Atlanta that she finally "grew up," recovering from the self-limited "disease" that is adolescence. (There's no cure for it, but if you give them enough time, the vast majority of them will outgrow it!) A few months ago, after a knock-down, drag-out fight with her boyfriend that split them apart for good, Nicole returned to Connecticut, moved back in with her father, and found herself a job. At our last visit, she seemed healthy, happy, and together. As her mother said when we first met, Nicole is smart and she "gets" it. I predict that from here on, because she will take care of herself, she will have few problems related to her porphyria.

Nicole's recent history underscores an important point: first and foremost, people with genetic disorders and birth defects are *people*. When I speak with families of children with Down syndrome, I take great pains to use this termi-nology: they are children first, children who happen to have Down syndrome; they are not *Down syndrome children,* a label that implies that everything they are is a consequence of the condition. Although this difference may seem subtle, it is vitally important.

CHAPTER 14

"Something's Bothering Me About This Baby"

I MET EDWIN RIVERA in the neonatal intensive care unit when he was four hours old. I'd been called to see him by Andy James, the neonatologist who was on call.

"I can't put my finger on it, Bob, but something's bothering me about this baby," Andy told me on the phone. "Something's not right, and I'm not sure what it is."

Coming from Andy, one of the best neonatologists I'd ever met, I knew this meant a lot. But frankly, looking down at Edwin lying in his Isolette, a small Plexiglas box with a mattress at the bottom, I had trouble understanding what it was that had so bothered the neonatologist. I couldn't find any good reason why a stat genetics consult had been requested for this baby.

Yes, Edwin was small; as Andy had mentioned over the phone, at 4 pounds, 11 ounces, he'd weighed a good 2 pounds less than what would have been expected for a newborn of his gestational age. But intrauterine growth restriction, the term for a birth weight significantly below expectation, had dozens of causes, only a few of which were genetic. And just watching him through the Plexiglas, I saw that Edwin, who was lying naked except for a disposable diaper, looked comfortable and was breathing at a normal rate without difficulty.

The infant's muscle tone also seemed appropriate for a full-term infant: he moved his perfectly formed arms and legs symmetrically, one side mirroring the other, as should be the case in a normal newborn. In addition, his head appeared to be of appropriate size, his dark hair was distributed in an appropriate pattern, his facial features were normally formed, and his neck and trunk looked great. So, at least superficially, except for his unexpectedly low weight, this baby seemed perfectly fine; watching him, I didn't get that feeling about which Andy James had been so bothered.

After a few minutes of watching Edwin through the Plexiglas, I opened the Isolette's door and formally examined him. The exam pretty much confirmed my initial impression: although small and thin, and with a slight hepatosplenomegaly (enlargement of his liver and spleen), the baby appeared to be a perfectly normal newborn.

As I was finishing my exam, Andy, who'd been on rounds when I'd arrived in the nursery, came to say hello. "Well, Bob, what do you think?" he asked. "Have you figured out what it is that's bothering me about this baby?"

Shaking my head, I replied, "Andy, I can't find much wrong with him. He is small, and he does have mild hepatosplenomegaly, but that's about all I can find."

"I don't know how to explain it," Andy said. "It's just a hunch; I just have the feeling that there's something really wrong with this kid, something that's not visible. Have you ever had that feeling about a patient?"

"Sure," I replied. "But to tell the truth, Andy, my abnormality detector isn't picking up any unusual signals around this baby." I went on to tell him that I thought the most likely explanation for Edwin's intrauterine growth restriction and liver and spleen enlargement was that the baby was suffering the effects of a congenital infection with one of the TORCH agents. TORCH is an acronym for a group of infectious agents—including toxoplasmosis, rubella, cytomegalovirus, and herpes (the "O" stands for *other*)—that is known to have the potential to infect the mother and cause harm to the developing embryo and fetus during pregnancy.

"I thought that, too," Andy said. "The only problem is, I spoke with the mother, and she said that except for the fact that they found that the baby wasn't growing well in the third trimester, this was a perfect pregnancy. She wasn't sick a single day in the nine months: she had no vomiting or diarrhea, no fever, no colds, and no rashes."

"Andy, you know that in a lot of cases, the infections that are the most devastating to the fetus cause pretty minor symptoms in the mother," I replied.

"I know, Bob, but as I said, in addition to that, there's just something about this baby that makes me uncomfortable. The lack of symptomatology in the mother just raises my suspicion more."

"Well, the fact that you're uncomfortable with this baby

means a lot to me," I said. "If you feel there's something wrong, there probably is. But other than a congenital infection, I can't think of anything helpful. I'd send off TORCH antibody tests and see what happens."

"We've already done it," the neonatologist responded. "Thanks for coming so fast."

"Sorry I couldn't be more helpful," I said as I went off to the nurses' station to write a consultation report in the baby's chart.

As I was finishing my note, Andy once again approached me. "I guess you're probably going to turn out to be right about an infection, Bob," he said. "I just got back the first set of blood tests on the baby. He's anemic and his bilirubin is already elevated. I'm going to have to start him on phototherapy."

I nodded. I knew that a deficiency of red blood cells (the cause of Edwin's anemia) is a feature of congenital infections, and that, because of damage to the liver, hepatitis may result, with its typical rise in the level of bilirubin. These lab results made me feel better about my assessment. I left the nursery feeling confident that I was right; I was pretty sure Edwin Rivera had a congenital infection.

HYPERBILIRUBINEMIA, THE BUILDUP of bilirubin in the blood, is a common problem in newborns. A by-product of the breakdown of red blood cells, a process that occurs throughout life, bilirubin is normally removed from the circulation by the action of the liver after it has gone through a process called conjugation. In neonates, the liver is not yet mature enough to produce the enzymes necessary for conjugating the circulating bilirubin; in most cases, it takes several days for the liver to start producing these proteins and to begin working. As a result, most babies pass through a brief period during which the sclerae (the whites of the eyes) may appear yellow and their skin may seem slightly jaundiced.

In 95 percent of cases, this transient hyperbilirubinemia and its resulting jaundice resolve without incident. In the remaining 5 percent, however—in babies who have complications such as prematurity, infections, or liver damage, or whose blood types are different from their mothers' (a condition called either ABO or Rh incompatibility)—the bilirubin reaches higher levels, raising concern that the chemical may cross the barrier that separates the blood from the central nervous system and cause a condition called kernicterus, which can result in permanent and irreparable brain damage.

When the level of bilirubin reaches into the range where concern about kernicterus exists, treatment to remove the chemical from the blood must be instituted. Two standard treatments exist to help lower the bilirubin level. First, the infant can undergo an exchange transfusion, a procedure in which the baby's blood is slowly removed in aliquots (fractional units) of 5 cubic centimeters, while donor blood is just as slowly introduced. Although capable of rapidly lowering the infant's bilirubin level, exchange transfusions are fraught with complications. Therefore, they are reserved for the most severe cases, the cases in which the hyperbilirubinemia is refractory to the more conservative method.

The second method, the one used as the first-line treatment, involves phototherapy, in which the baby is placed under banks of fluorescent lights. Under these lights, a chemical reaction occurs in the skin that transforms bilirubin into a substance called lumirubin, a compound that can more easily be eliminated from the bloodstream. Although this reaction occurs slowly and the net effect is a gradual decrease in bilirubin level, phototherapy, which causes no long-term adverse effects, is usually enough to produce resolution of the problem.

And so, on his first day of life, when Edwin Rivera was found to have an elevation in the level of bilirubin in his blood, Andy James placed the infant under a double bank of fluorescent bili lights and ordered that a repeat level be obtained in eight hours. The treatment worked: the repeat bilirubin level, drawn when the infant was 16 hours old, was no higher than the first. And the third level, taken the next morning when Edwin was 24 hours old, showed a decline. It seemed as if Andy's plan had worked: kernicterus was not going to be a problem with Edwin Rivera.

But while Edwin's bilirubin level was stabilizing, a spectacular new problem arose.

That next morning I was greeted by a phone call from Andy James. "Bob, the baby with intrauterine growth restriction has developed the weirdest rash I've ever seen. He's got blisters all over his body."

"Blisters?" I asked. "That is weird. I know babies with congenital infections can have lots of different rashes, but I've never heard of blisters. How big are they?"

"Huge," he replied. "And when you rub them, they weep clear fluid. I've never seen anything like it before."

I told him I'd be right over. And since I'm not very good at rashes, I also asked if he'd called for help from a dermatologist.

"I already thought of that," he replied. "Suzanne Cummings is on her way. You'll probably get here at around the same time."

As it turned out, I reached the NICU a few minutes before Suzanne, one of our hospital's best dermatologists. Looking through the Isolette's Plexiglas, I was amazed by what I saw: Edwin, the happy, satisfied baby I'd seen the day before, had been replaced by a crying, miserable wretch whose skin was covered from his forehead to the soles of his feet with large, swollen, apparently painful blisters. As I stared at the baby, Andy approached and said, "Have you ever seen anything like this before?"

I had actually seen something like this before, in a baby who had a disease called epidermolysis bullosa (EB), a rare inherited disorder in which the skin forms blisters at sites of trauma. But newborns with EB differed in at least two ways from what we were seeing in Edwin. First, those babies were usually born with blisters. And second, in EB, blisters didn't occur indiscriminately all over the body; they occurred only in areas of irritation.

I was explaining these differences to Andy when Suzanne Cummings entered the nursery. After saying hello, she looked down at the baby and uttered only two words: "Oh my." Silently, she donned a pair of gloves and, after opening the door of the Isolette, she very gingerly began examining Edwin. As Andy had mentioned, a clear, colorless liquid emerged from each blister that was touched. "Bullae from head to toe," Suzanne muttered, adding, "amazing. When did they appear?"

"Last night," Andy responded, "when the baby was about eight hours old."

"These are bili lights?" she asked, pointing toward the

fluorescent bulbs. After we nodded, the dermatologist asked, "When did you start phototherapy?"

"At about five o'clock yesterday afternoon," Andy answered.

"A few hours before the bullae appeared?" she asked.

Again, Andy nodded.

At that point, Suzanne peeled back the tapes that held the infant's diaper in place, exposing Edwin's perineum; the whole area, from waistline to scrotum, was completely free of bullae. While the dermatologist nodded her head, Andy and I turned and looked at each other, our eyes wide as saucers.

Next, using only the tips of her fingers, Suzanne lifted the baby's right shoulder off the mattress. The maneuver was obviously painful for the baby; his screaming crescendoed as the dermatologist applied her fingers to the blistered skin. But when the shoulder was off the mattress, we saw another unexpected sight: Edwin's back was also completely free of the rash. "Amazing," the dermatologist uttered for the second time that morning.

I had no idea what had caused these findings, no explanation for why some areas of Edwin's skin were so badly damaged while others were completely free of lesions.

But Suzanne Cummings already knew the answer. "Andy," she asked, "is there someplace dark around here? Someplace that gets no sunlight?" After thinking for a few seconds, Andy pointed to the unit's storage closet.

Without hesitation, Suzanne slid her gloved hand below Edwin's rump and, after carefully lifting the baby's butt off the mattress, removed his diaper from the Isolette. After stopping at the nurses' station to grab her bag, Suzanne followed Andy into the storage closet. I brought up the rear.

As she pulled a small lamp from her bag, Suzanne said, "I don't want to say anything yet, because I'm not sure if I'm right. The distribution of the lesions is unusual: the bullae appear only in areas where the skin has been exposed to the photo-therapy light. I know of only one disorder that causes anything like that. Bob, would you close the door?"

I pulled the door of the supply closet shut, and the room became pitch black.

"This is my Wood's lamp," the dermatologist continued. "I'm going to turn it on now. Watch closely."

In a matter of seconds, an eerie purplish light began to emanate from the lamp Suzanne was holding in her left hand. Simultaneously, from the diaper, which the dermatologist was holding in her right hand, a bright bluish red pigment seemed to appear. "See the glow?" Suzanne asked. "That proves it: this baby has congenital erythropoietic porphyria. Amazing."

CONGENITAL ERYTHROPOIETIC PORPHYRIA (CEP) is a rare form of porphyria, part of the same group of disorders that affected Nicole Ludlow. As in acute intermittent porphyria (AIP), the deficiency of a single enzyme necessary for the pro-duction of heme leads to a series of symptoms and signs related to both a deficiency of heme (and a resulting deficiency in both hemoglobin and red blood cells) and a buildup in the blood-stream of toxic precursors in the biosynthetic pathway. In AIP, medical problems include anemia and intermittent neurologic and psychiatric symptoms, the kinds of problems that have plagued Nicole Ludlow all her life. But individuals with CEP also suffer from anemia more severe than the form that occurs in AIP, causing affected individuals to require periodic blood transfusions for survival; also, the buildup of the precursor porphyrins have far more severe and constant effects. Red in color, the porphyrins that are present in the blood of individuals with CEP are photosensitive: when exposed to any kind of light, these chemicals are toxic to the skin. In the presence of light, the chemicals produce blisters on the skin like the ones that formed on Edwin's face, trunk, and limbs soon after he began receiving phototherapy; the blisters ultimately heal to form scars. After repeated exposure to light, people with CEP become more and more disfigured: their skin becomes covered with scars, and some areas on their scalp lack hair whereas some areas on their skin sprout hair indiscriminately.

Interestingly, it is the presence of these clinical features that has led some medical historians to speculate that individuals with CEP served as the origin of the legend of the vampire, an ancient myth that is present in a large number of diverse cultures. Vampires are portrayed as deceased individuals who find themselves rejected by the hallowed earth of cemeteries because they have been cursed in some way. Unable to achieve a state of peace in their own graves, they metamorphosize into the undead or the living dead, trapped between the worlds of the living and the dead. Hideously ugly and constantly in need of sustenance, vampires are destined to walk the earth after dark, looking to feed on the blood of the innocent.

Now consider individuals with CEP. Because the porphyrins in their bloodstream result in photosensitivity, these people's faces are scarred. And because of the photosensitivity, coupled with their psychological sensitivity, they learn early in life to leave their homes only at night. Finally, because of the deposition of the abnormal red porphyrins in the structure of their teeth, people with CEP develop erythrodontia (literally, "red teeth"), giving the uninformed the impression that they have been drinking blood. It's not difficult to understand how, in an age when superstition and ignorance ruled, the birth of an infant with CEP might have led to the beginning of a tale of the undead that ultimately grew into today's legend.

THE ELEVATED LEVEL of porphyrins in Edwin Rivera's bloodstream had led to an excessive amount of the chemical compounds being excreted in his urine. It was this phenomenon that caused his diaper to glow, a finding that had confirmed his diagnosis: Suzanne knew Edwin had CEP because the baby's urine was packed with fluorescent red chemicals.

After leaving the supply closet, Andy walked over to Edwin's Isolette and switched off the bili lights. Taking a clean sheet from the NICU's laundry cart, he covered the Isolette's Plexiglas so that none of the room's ambient light could reach the baby.

"This explains why he's so anemic," I said to Suzanne as she wrote her consult note in Edwin's chart. "And I guess the enlargement of his liver and spleen is the result of extramedullary hematopoiesis [essentially, his body's attempt to make as many blood cells as possible, using blood-forming sites other than the usual bone marrow]. But why is he so growth-retarded? That doesn't make sense."

The dermatologist shrugged her shoulders. Edwin's growth retardation didn't make sense to any of us then, and it still doesn't. But further testing proved that Suzanne was correct: a test of Edwin's blood revealed absence of uroporphyrinogen III cosynthase, the enzyme whose deficiency is responsible for CEP.

AFTER ANDY COVERED his Isolette with the sheet, Edwin remained like that, in the dark, in a corner of the NICU, for nearly four months. During this time, the boy's parents, who initially had a difficult time coming to grips with the nature and severity of their son's problem, and the implications it had for his and their future, learned how to take care of him. Eventually, they took him home to a life in near total darkness.

Today, at age three, Edwin has a number of serious problems. He continues to live in the dark, cut off from all light, venturing out of the family's apartment only after nightfall. He's been chronically ill: as predicted in the newborn period, because of his severe anemia, he's come to rely on periodic blood transfusions, which are administered during overnight stays in the infants' unit at the Children's Hospital. For reasons that are not fully understood, he has frequent serious infections, many of which require long stays in the hospital for intravenous antibiotic therapy (of course, when starting IV lines in him, the resident performing the procedure has to work in the dark). To say the least, the boy's life (as well as the lives of his parents) has not been easy.

It's never difficult to figure out when Edwin has been admitted to the hospital: he's the one in the room in which the shades have been drawn, the lights have been turned out, and the light switch has been taped into the off position. In his hospital crib,

Edwin lies behind an orange Plexiglas sheet that blocks out most of the wavelengths of light that would prove most harmful to his skin. Because of the careful precautions taken by his parents, Edwin's skin is not terribly scarred at this point. But how can a child live like this? How can he grow and develop, make friends, go to school, and live in society with a condition that allows him to exist outside his home only in the dark?

Sadly, I'm not too optimistic about Edwin's future. Only a bone marrow transplant will free him from his nocturnal existence. Although this procedure—which replace his own bone marrow cells (which lack the enzyme needed to produce heme) with donor cells that can produce the required enzyme—could free him from this restrictive existence, there are some serious problems: first, bone marrow transplantation carries with it a 20 percent mortality rate, a risk that Edwin's parents are not yet ready to accept. Second, for the procedure to have the best chance of succeeding, a suitable donor must be found; because Edwin has had so many blood transfusions in his short life, transfusions that have come from multiple donors, his system has produced antibodies to the blood of virtually everyone on earth. Thus far, no match has been found. And Edwin's problems continue.

Since Edwin's birth, whenever I see Andy James, I think of the uneasy feeling he had in the hours after the infant's arrival in the NICU. I'm still not sure what it was about the baby that triggered that response in the neonatologist, but I am sure of one thing: now, whenever he calls and says "Bob, something's bothering me about this baby," I take that concern very, very seriously.

Postscript

EDWIN CONTINUED TO HAUNT the infants' unit for more than a year; his infections had become so frequent that he was virtually always hospitalized, spending weeks in the hospital for every day he was at home. He essentially lived in a darkened room on the ward, lying in the crib behind his orange Plexiglas sheet.

And then, one day Edwin was gone.

I didn't notice it at first. I guess I realized that he'd been discharged, but I must have figured that he had recovered from one infection or another and had been sent home. As time passed, I was too busy to realize that he had been absent from the unit for longer than I would have expected. And then I kind of just forgot about him.

An entire year passed. It was one of the first nice days of spring: the sun was out, the temperature was in the seventies, and I was out on the sidewalk in front of the hospital, breathing the fresh air when I saw Edwin's mother. She was walking hand-in-hand with a little boy, who I guessed was three or four years old. It took me a few seconds to realize that this little boy was Edwin.

He was out in the sunlight; he was dressed like everyone else on the sidewalk, in a short-sleeve shirt and a pair of jeans. His face, though showing some of the scars that resulted from his disease, was not covered with any unusual protection from the sun. He looked like a normal kid.

I guess Edwin's mother read the quizzical look on my face, because she said, "Yes, Dr. Marion, it is Edwin. It is a miracle, isn't it?"

"What happened?" was all I managed to get out.

"A miracle," she said again. "After he was discharged from here, we took him to Memorial Sloan-Kettering. They gave Edwin a bone marrow transplant."

"Whose bone marrow did they use?" I asked.

"Mine," she replied. "It wasn't a perfect match, but after he had been so sick for so long, my husband and I, we figured it was worth a try, that it might make him better than the way he was. Believe me, Dr. Marion, after he got my bone marrow, he was sick for months, in and out of the ICU there. He had every complication you could think of; a few times, we thought we were going to lose him. But then, one day, he just started to get better. And here he is."

And there he was: at four years old, out on the street in the sun, looking healthy and happy, a little the worse for the wear, but acting like any other four-year-old. For sure, a miracle.

I don't know what Edwin's future will be, whether his bone marrow will behave itself or whether he will reject it (or whether it will reject him, a complication known as a graft-versus-host reaction). But at least for now, by manipulating his bone marrow, the doctors have "cured" his genetic disorder — his mother's cells (which, because she is an obligate carrier, produce only 50 percent of the normal amount of the enzyme missing from Edwin's cells) having replaced his mutated cells. When I began my career in clinical genetics, such an outcome was only a dream; now it is an everyday occurrence. What a great time it is to be in this field!

CHAPTER 15

Two Miracles, One Year Later

O NE LATE MORNING on a Friday in November, I'd just walked through the door leading to the inpatient unit at Garwood Children's Hospital. Coming at me at what seemed like 40 miles per hour, bearing down like a cruise missile homing in on its target, was a little red tricycle. Steering and peddling that tricycle was my patient Clarence Aguirre. Barbara, Clarence's physical therapist, who was running alongside, ordered the boy to stop: "Clarence, you don't want to run down Dr. Marion, do you?" Complying, Clarence brought the missile to a halt a few inches from my feet.

Clearly proud of himself, Clarence flashed his devilish grin (he was missing his two front teeth, which made his smile more distinctive); the little guy, then a few months shy of his third birthday, was strapped onto the seat of the tricycle; his feet had been Velcroed to the pedals, and his hands had been strapped to the handlebar. Taking it all in, I also began to smile.

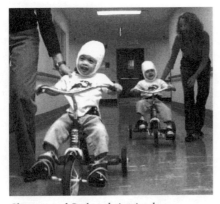

Clarence and Carl on their tricycles, November 2004

This was the latest in what was a growing list of miracles accomplished by the amazing Aguirre twins.

Miracle was a word that was used a lot when speaking of these brothers. Delivered by cesarean section in Manila, the Philippines, on April 19, 2002, Carl and Clarence were the first children born to their mother, Arlene. During a routine sonogram performed when she was in her third month of pregnancy, Arlene, who worked as a nurse for a large corporation in Manila, had learned that she was carrying craniopagus conjoined twins, twin boys who had developed separately and perfectly in all ways except for one: through a chance occurrence, a 1-in-10-million error in the process of forming as monozygotic or identical twins, the two genetically identical embryos had failed to separate in the region of the apex of their skulls.

This relatively tiny embryonic flaw would have a huge impact in the twins' extrauterine lives, because—as was immediately apparent to Arlene, her doctors, and her family—these boys, although healthy at birth, would never be able to survive the way they were. Because of their head-to-head fusion, Carl and Clarence would never be able to sit, stand, or walk; unless something was done, they would spend their lives lying on their backs or on their sides. Arlene understood from the beginning that if they were not separated, the boys would die of aspiration pneumonia, an inability to eat, or a combination of the two during the first years of their lives.

But how could they be separated? In 2002, not a single set of craniopagus conjoined twins had ever been successfully separated. And even if surgery could be performed, how could Arlene—who, following the birth of her sons, had lost her nursing job and moved back to her parents' home on the rural island of Negros—ever be able to find a neurosurgeon who might be willing to perform such a risky and unproven operation? And as a single mother with little money, how could she pay for an operation even if she could find someone to do it? The situation seemed impossible.

But sometimes, through persistence, hard work, and determination, the impossible becomes possible. Arlene persevered; with the assistance of the boys' pediatrician and a local social worker, and by working the Internet, she pursued every lead that might put her in contact with anyone who might be able to help. Through a series of improbable connections involving international children's aid agencies, interested private parties, and just dumb luck, the plight of Carl and Clarence came to the attention of Dr. James Goodrich, chief of pediatric neurosurgery at Children's Hospital. Although Dr. Goodrich had, during his distinguished 20-plus-year career, amassed a great deal of experience repairing complex congenital malformation of the skull and face, he had never before performed surgery on a set of conjoined twins. But after studying the photographs and the preliminary CAT scans and MRIs that had been performed in Manila (which indicated that although the boys shared skull, meninges, the membranous covering of the brain, and a tangle of arteries and veins, their brains appeared to be completely separate), and after a great deal of discussion with colleagues both in the Bronx and throughout the world, Dr. Goodrich concluded that he might be able to help the Aguirre twins.

The medical literature didn't support Dr. Goodrich's conclusion. At that time, in every case in which separation of craniopagus twins had been attempted, one or both twins had either died or suffered serious brain damage during or soon after the surgery. Dr. Goodrich's optimism, though, was based on the fact that he believed he could identify the flaw in the surgical planning that had led to these failures. In the past, all attempts at separating craniopagus twins had been performed in a single marathon session, operations that lasted 70 hours or more. Dr. Goodrich reasoned that there were three major problems caused by this strategy: first, the stress placed on the circulatory systems of the patients by such lengthy periods of anesthesia is immense, making them less-than-optimal surgical candidates; second, the long hours required teams of surgeons, and in team surgery the adage that a chain is only as strong as its weakest link really is true; and third, and most important, experience had shown that the marathon procedure approach repeatedly led to difficulties near the end of the operation because of problems caused by the separation of shared blood vessels. Basically, as blood vessels shared between the twins were separated, the remaining vessels became larger, carrying an increasing percentage of the common blood supply between the twins' brains. Eventually, what had been believed to be a small and inconsequential vein or artery at the beginning of the procedure became a gushing torrent of blood near the end. This made it almost impossible to perform the final separation without the loss of a tremendous amount of blood, a consequence that led to both brains becoming oxygen deficient.

Not only had Dr. Goodrich discovered this flaw, but he also believed that he had developed a solution. His plan was based on his experience in performing hundreds of operations that corrected complicated craniofacial malformations. In providing surgical care to patients like A.C. Sheridan, Dr. Goodrich had learned that it was not necessary to repair everything at once and that, in fact, a single operation was actually contraindicated in many cases. Repairs could be performed as a series of staged procedures, individually designed to address each child's underlying problem. If staged procedure proved successful in the repair of other craniofacial malformations, why couldn't it also be applied to the separation of conjoined twins?

Goodrich's plan was to separate Carl and Clarence Aguirre in stages, in a series of four or five short operations, during each of which a little more of the boys' shared skull, meninges, and blood vessels would be divided. Between procedures, as the twins continued to live their attached lives, they would have time to recover from the previous surgery, gain the strength needed to undergo the next, and, most important, give their blood vessels the chance to adjust to the slow separation by developing what are called collateral vessels, thus preventing the complications faced in the past by surgeons nearing the end of marathon separation surgeries.

To those of us consulted by Dr. Goodrich, the plan made tremendous sense. Considering that we all agreed that the twins would not be able to survive for very long the way they were, it seemed to be worth a try, the only real shot these boys had to survive. So Dr. Goodrich set about convincing the administrative staffs at both Children's Hospital and at Garwood Children's Hospital, the pediatric rehab hospital in Westchester County where he thought the boys could recuperate between operations, that they should eat all costs incurred. Dr. Goodrich, an excellent salesman, quickly succeeded in reaching his goal. The Montefiore Medical Center, the large voluntary hospital that operates our Children's Hospital, would underwrite the surgical and medical care the boys received and Garwood would serve as home base for Carl and Clarence and Arlene, the place they'd live and receive therapy both before and after separation.

And so on September 10, 2003, after months of painstaking planning, Arlene arrived with Carl and Clarence, then 17 months old, at Kennedy International Airport in New York. After deplaning, the boys and Arlene were transported to Garwood, where they immediately began to settle in.

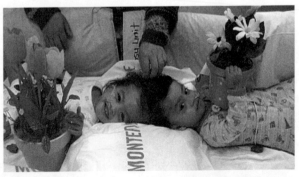

Clarence (left) and Carl, soon after their arrival in New York

That's when I first met the Aguirres. As the geneticist at Garwood and the director of genetics at the Children's Hospital, I was the logical person to provide and coordinate the continuing medical care the boys would need during the months ahead. Even though I had seen numerous pictures of them in the weeks prior to their arrival, I had trouble believing what I was seeing when I first laid eyes on the two boys. Seeing photos is one thing; viewing two otherwise completely normal toddlers, perfectly formed in every way except one, moving and playing and interacting with their mother and staff members, but fixed together at the head, is quite another. Watching them in real time caused my jaw to drop and made my knees go a little weak. Once I adjusted to what I was seeing, however, I quickly came to understand that Carl and Clarence were two very sick little boys.

They were severely malnourished: at 17 months, they weighed less than half of what twins of that age should weigh. Typical 17-month-old children should be able to sit up and stand, and walk forward and backward; the position Carl and Clarence were in prevented them from being able to do any of these things. Also, they had additional huge medical issues: during their initial exam, Clarence, the smaller of the twins, was noted to have a blood pressure of 220/150, dangerously high for a child of that age (or, in fact, for a human of any age); Carl, the larger and more placid twin, had blood pressure that was in the low normal range. Also, because of the problem caused by their position, each boy had essentially lived for 17 months feeding in a lying-down posture; a small amount of formula was a constant presence in their mouths, which had caused each of them to develop multiple cavities, a problem that, following cranial surgery, could predispose them to a serious infection. Before any attempts at surgical separation could be attempted, the boys needed to be fattened up, Clarence's hypertension needed to be controlled, and their teeth needed to be attended to.

Something else was perfectly clear from early on: the twins had personalities that were as different as night and day. Outgoing and friendly, Clarence was perpetually happy, with a smile that could light up a room. Quieter and more thoughtful, Carl was more cautious about letting outsiders see his smile. As we worked through the initial evaluations, each member of the group of specialists who would ultimately come to be known as Team Aguirre wondered how two genetically identical infants (DNA testing had been done on cells obtained from their skin) who had been reared in exactly the same environment could have turned out so different. (Thank goodness they enjoyed watching the same TV shows; from their first hours in New York, Carl and Clarence fell in love with *The Wiggles;* while watching the show on TV, the twins seemed mesmerized.)

There were other things about Carl and Clarence that we didn't understand. Although we could explain why their motor development was delayed, their conjoinedness should not have affected their cognitive development. Yet, when they arrived in New York, neither boy spoke even a single word. Why weren't they speaking? Was there something about their brains that prevented them from reaching cognitive milestones?

And what was it that was causing Clarence's blood pressure to be that high? Could their connectedness be the cause?

(This became more of a puzzle after we began treating Clarence with antihypertensive medications; although we knew the boys shared a common blood supply, the medications, which eventually brought Clarence's blood pressure under control, had no effect on Carl.) Although answering these questions would play no role in their separation, the curiosity of our team members needed to be satisfied.

FOLLOWING THEIR ARRIVAL, we worked on solving each of the boys' health issues. Via nasogastric tubes, we began pumping high-calorie formula into their stomachs around the clock. After a workup to detect the cause of his hypertension proved negative, Clarence was begun on medication; ultimately, it took four drugs to bring his blood pressure into anything resembling a range acceptable for surgery. Finally, to prevent the possibility of infection following the first operation, the twins saw the dentist, who extracted multiple cavity-riddled baby teeth.

While their medical problems were being fixed, Dr. Goodrich and his team of surgeons planned out how they would go about separating the two boys. We already knew (and MRIs of the boys' heads done at the Children's Hospital confirmed) that, in addition to scalp, skull, and meninges, the boys were held together by a tangle of veins that returned the brain's blood supply to the heart and arteries that brought blood to their brains. A magnetic resonance arteriogram (MRA) demonstrated that these vessels actually "belonged" to Clarence (i.e., they had developed from his circulatory system); he essentially was the drainage system for Carl's cerebral blood supply.

We later came to understand that Clarence was also pumping blood into Carl's cerebral circulation, and that this was actually the cause of Clarence's hypertension (he needed to generate more pressure to reach his brother's brain). It was also the cause of his small size (because of his role as the "pump twin," Clarence was burning more calories than his brother), and it explained why Carl had a laid-back personality (it was related to the relatively low flow of blood to his brain).

The problem posed to the surgeons was how to separate the connecting blood vessels while providing a way for Carl's cerebral blood to return to his heart. As already mentioned, Dr. Goodrich's solution to this problem was to perform a series of short procedures. During each operation, he and his surgical partner, Dr. David Staffenberg, our director of craniofacial plastic surgery, would remove a small portion of the joined skull and divide the joined blood vessels that lay beneath this section of skull. After the allotted portion was separated, the skull would be closed and the boys would return to Garwood, where they would recover from the surgery; continue receiving physical, occupational, and speech therapy; continue gaining weight; and prepare for the next procedure. Dr. Goodrich hoped that such an approach would "force" Carl to develop a series of collateral vessels that would ultimately form his own personal cerebral blood drainage system. The surgeons believed it would take at least four operations before the final separation could be attempted.

THE FIRST OPERATION took place on October 13, 2003, a little over a month after the twins first arrived in New York. The boys were transferred from Garwood and taken to the operating room (OR), where they were placed on a specially designed table. Then the surgeons went to work. Like astronauts taking their first steps on the lunar surface, Drs. Goodrich and Staffenberg removed a block of skull from the frontal region of the boys' joined skull and tentatively began exploring the region. As had been predicted by the imaging studies, the brains appeared perfectly formed and separate. There were virtually no joined blood vessels in this region; when such a shared vein was encountered, Dr. Goodrich would tie it off with suture material and wait; if no enlargement of surrounding vessels occurred, if everything in the vascular bed remained calm, he would tie a second knot and clip the vessel between the two knots. This first procedure, which lasted just over two hours, went without a hitch; at no point did the surgeons or anesthesiologist encounter any problems or have any concerns about the safety of the boys.

After the procedure ended, the boys were brought to the intensive care unit on the top floor of the hospital—Children's Hospital at Montefiore (CHAM) 10—where they bounced back from the procedure extremely quickly. Within 24 hours, they were essentially back to their pre-surgical selves. On the third day after surgery, once all of us on the medical side of their care were convinced that no post-op complications had occurred, the boys were shipped back to Garwood via ambulance. The ground had been broken; based on the results, Team Aguirre was optimistic that we were both on our way to making history, and more important, to providing the twins with a shot at leading a normal life.

BACK AT GARWOOD, Carl and Clarence continued to do well: their wound healed, they gained weight, and they continued to make developmental strides. Within a month, we felt that they were already in good enough condition to undergo a second procedure.

And so, on November 23, they were transferred back to CHAM and brought to the OR. During this second operation, the surgeons extended the cut they'd made into the frontal region of the shared skull laterally so that approximately one-third of the skull was now divided. This procedure, which lasted for four hours, also went off without a single complication. Again within three days, Carl and Clarence returned to Garwood. They returned to the Bronx on February 20 for the third stage of the separation, a procedure that lasted for nearly five hours, during which the skull was divided laterally on the other side from the frontal region. By the end of this third operation, the surgeons estimated that the skull was 90 percent separated, being held in place by surgical screws and wires. Although the vast majority of the skull and meninges had been divided, Drs. Goodrich and Staffenberg understood that the final stage of the separation would be the most difficult. In the back, or occipital, region of the shared skull—the only remaining section that had not yet been separated—the boys shared a large plexus of blood vessels; it would take hours of painstaking surgery to successfully separate all of these vessels.

Meanwhile, though, the twins continued to thrive. At Garwood, they had managed to put some meat on their bones. Amazingly, following each surgical procedure, Clarence's hypertension had become easier to control: with the separation of

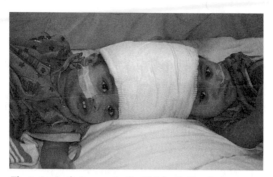

The twins in their room in the Children's Hospital at Montefiore ICU, following the second procedure

more vessels, it took fewer medications to keep his blood pressure in a normal range. And with the help of their therapists, the boys' trunk and limb muscles were becoming stronger. They were healthy, they seemed happy, and with each day they were more alert and active. As the winter of 2004 turned to spring, around the time Carl and Clarence celebrated their second birthday, the time for the final separation was drawing near.

But before Dr. Goodrich and his team would perform that final separation surgery, the twins needed to prove to all of us that they could survive independently. In July 2004, in order to see whether Carl had developed his own venous system, the MRA test was repeated. This study showed exactly what we'd hoped it would: deep within Carl's brain, where there previously had been no blood vessels evident, a tangle of small wormlike squiggles had appeared. Dr. Goodrich's theory had been correct: through the use of tiny collateral vessels, Carl had "built" his own system of venous return from the cerebral circulation. That MRA told us that the time to separate Carl from Clarence had arrived.

EARLY ON THE MORNING of August 4, 2004, the twins were lifted onto a gurney. The boys, who'd arrived at CHAM 10 from Garwood the night before, had already been intubated (i.e., a tube had been passed through each nose, down through the pharynx, through the vocal cords and into the trachea; these tubes would allow the anesthesiologists to breathe for them during the surgery). While the gurney was pushed from the ICU toward the operating suite, a caravan of people followed close behind. There was Arlene, who had not slept for days. There were people from Garwood, including the boys' social worker and a few of their therapists. I was also tagging along. During the long day that lay ahead, I would serve as a medical liaison for Arlene, an interpreter who would be communicating with the surgical team and translating to the boys' mom exactly what was going on in the OR.

While our group settled into a room in the pediatric day hospital, the twins were transferred from the gurney onto the special operating table that had been fabricated for them, their heads overlying a region that could, at just the right moment, pivot apart, splitting the table into two. After the twins were settled, the anesthesia team and the surgeons made their final preparations.

To those of us in the waiting room, time passed unbearably slowly and the tension was fierce; we tried to keep Arlene's mind off what was happening a few feet away, but it was impossible. As the hours passed, we were desperate for news from the OR, but with the surgeons so busy, reports were infrequent.

Meanwhile, in the lobby of Children's Hospital, dozens of reporters from TV, radio, and newspaper outlets from around the world had also begun to settle in. By this time the story of the conjoined twins from the Philippines was big news, the boys' progress having been covered for months on NBC's *Dateline*, in newspapers, and elsewhere.

At 9:00 A.M., with everything ready, Dr. Staffenberg made his first incision. Soon Dr. Goodrich was wading through the occipital region of the shared skull, finding and meticulously dividing the remaining vessels that held the boys together. The work was close, painstaking, demanding, and extremely time-consuming.

At 4:30 P.M., a major hurdle was passed. After assessing the situation, the surgical team decided that the boys' conditions were good enough to proceed to the final separation. Prior to this time, the opportunity had always existed to turn back, to end the procedure, a decision that would leave Carl and Clarence alive but needing to continue to exist in their joined state. But now that the decision had been made to proceed, there could be no turning back: too much separation had been accomplished to quit. Dr. Goodrich came out to inform Arlene of the plan. Immediately, as the realization hit that this was it, the anxiety level in the waiting room ratcheted up a little further.

While Dr. Goodrich was speaking with us, the hospital's public affairs department issued a press release announcing that the surgeons were proceeding with the final separation. The media representatives camped out in CHAM's lobby, starved for any information from the surgical team, immediately transmitted this news to the world.

In the OR, the surgery was proceeding as planned. Sure, things were moving ahead slowly; certainly, the anxiety was nearly unbearable. But the bottom line was that Carl and Clarence were weathering the surgical storm without any complications. Things were looking up.

But then, at around 7:00 P.M., out of the clear blue, the surgeons stumbled onto a problem that no one had anticipated.

While continuing to work his way through the dissection of the tangle of conjoined blood vessels, Dr. Goodrich encountered a portion of cerebral cortex that would not separate. In spite of all the preparations, despite all the CAT scans and MRIs and MRAs that had led up to this moment, it became apparent that a portion of what we all thought were two separate brains was actually fused together. Now, Dr. Goodrich is not a man who panics, but for the first time since the Aguirres had arrived in New York, he was not exactly sure how to proceed: cutting through a conjoined section of brain could have serious consequences for one or both twins. An injury to the brain of Carl or Clarence (or both), even one that was intentionally made by the knife of the surgeon, could cause seizures, cognitive or motor impairment, bleeding, or even death. So Dr. Goodrich had to decide what to do. Should he stop here, admitting that the separation was not feasible, and simply close up the joined skulls? After so much had already been separated, was this even an option? He wasn't sure; he needed to do some thinking.

The surgery came to a halt. The surgeons called the neuroradiologists, and together they went over every imaging study that had been done since the twins had been born. They looked at cut after cut, photo after photo; in none of them could anyone identify any sign of conjoined cortices. Yet, amazingly, there the boys were in the operating room, with two brains that communicated in a 0.5-centimeter knuckle of connection!

After nearly two hours of contemplation, realizing that the surgery had progressed too far to turn back, Dr. Goodrich decided to move ahead with the separation. He would tease apart the joined section along a tiny indentation in the shared region, a spot that looked to him like it might have been a natural cleavage plane. After the decision was made, the operation proceeded.

Back in the waiting room, none of us had any idea of the crisis that had developed in the OR. It was only later, after the procedure had ended, that the surgeons shared this information. Both Drs. Goodrich and Staffenberg understood what such news would mean to Arlene.

Once the decision to proceed was reached and the operation began again, the surgeons made rapid progress. At a few minutes before 11:00 P.M., the team accomplished the first phase of this operation's goals. With all bridging vessels now successfully divided, it was time to separate Carl from Clarence.

On Dr. Goodrich's signal, the table was pivoted apart.

For the first time in their lives, the boys were now lying on separate tables, about a foot apart from each other.

At the site of this, the OR team broke into cheers.

Minutes later, with a mixture of weariness and exhilaration, Dr. Staffenberg left the OR and walked to the waiting room. Arlene and the rest of us took a collective breath at his appearance.

"Arlene," Dr. Staffenberg said, with words he'd rehearsed for months by this time, "I'm happy to tell you that you've got two separate sons!"

His announcement was followed by a scream from Arlene. The room filled with jubilation. We began a group hug; we all had tears in our eyes as we hugged and kissed and held on to one another. Cell phones and cameras appeared, and the happy news was spread throughout the extended family that had developed around Arlene since the family's arrival in New York.

Nearly immediately, the waiting room's TV, tuned to the local news, broke into a story with the following announcement: "Doctors at the Children's Hospital at Montefiore have now successfully separated the Aguirre twins!"

The impossible had been accomplished.

THE FORMAL SEPARATION of Carl and Clarence was not the end of this marathon procedure: before they could leave the OR, the boys' brains needed to be covered with meninges and skin. The surgeons broke into two teams, with Dr. Goodrich leading the group working on Carl, while Dr. Staffenberg took the lead in closing Clarence's head. Because the meninges that existed actually belonged to Clarence, the surgeons used an artificial membrane, manufactured from pig omentum, to cover Carl's skull. By 2:30 A.M., 18 ½ hours after the surgery had begun, the work was done. Tenderly, the boys were transferred by the OR staff onto separate gurneys. With exuberant members of the surgical team by their side, accompanied by a video crew from NBC, the twins took their first trip as separate beings. Out of the OR, down the hall, they passed through a set of double doors. On the other side of those doors, an exhausted Arlene stood, waiting with tears in her eyes for her first glimpse of her separate sons.

She hugged them; she kissed them. Her dream had become

a reality: the boys were separate. But their journey was far from complete.

ALTHOUGH THE TWINS spent three weeks in the pediatric ICU, their post-op course was free of complication. They awoke from the anesthesia no worse for the wear. At no time did they need any special intervention.

The story of the twins' separation was front-page news around the world. In the days following the surgery, thousands of e-mails poured into the Children's Hospital. When she wasn't standing over the ICU beds of her two sons, a relieved Arlene spent most of her free time reading these e-mails; she vowed to answer every one.

All of us who were involved with the twins wondered what the boys' immediate reaction would be when they awoke from their anesthetically induced sleep to discover that they were no longer joined. We imagined that this would be a stunning revelatory moment for them, an instant during which they recognized their separateness. Would they respond with shock and horror, like a man waking to find that his arm or leg had been amputated? Or would they be happy and relieved, like a patient whose massive tumor had been removed and found to be benign? As the anesthesia lightened, we watched to see exactly what would happen when they opened their eyes.

About 70 hours after they arrived in the OR, after Dr. Goodrich decided it was finally safe to allow them to wake up, the moment arrived. What a letdown! Neither twin registered any kind of reaction. Upon opening their eyes, Carl and Clarence looked at the child lying in the adjacent hospital bed, and seemed not to recognize who that other child was! I guess this shouldn't have been that surprising to us; after all, because of the way they'd been joined, neither boy had ever really seen the other before that moment. Carl and Clarence seemed to assume that the child in the next bed was just some other kid who'd been plunked down beside them, like one of their classmates in the preschool classes at Garwood. Oh well, so much for drama!

ON AUGUST 30, the boys left CHAM. With Arlene pushing them in a twin stroller, and with their doctors at their sides, the boys passed through the main entrance of the Children's Hospital; were met by cheering media, staff members, and passersby; and loaded into two separate ambulances. With sirens blaring, the ambulances headed off, back toward Garwood, where Carl and Clarence would continue their rehabilitation.

THEIR DISCHARGE FROM the ICU at CHAM marked the end of one stage of the twins' lives and the start of the next. It was time for Carl and Clarence to try to become like other sets of twins. As opposed to the rapidity with which the surgery had wrought its changes, the rehabilitation of the boys was going to be a long and arduous process.

Back at Garwood, the twins resumed their rigorous therapy schedules. But their lives were different now: they slept in separate beds, played with separate toys, watched different TV shows on their separate TV sets. And to some extent, following their separation surgery, even their personalities underwent something of a transformation. This change was most dramatically seen in Carl.

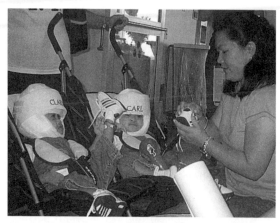

Clarence and Carl, on the morning they left CHAM. The names on the front of their surgical bandage were suggested by Nadine Staffenberg (Dr. David's wife), in response to our concerns that, following separation, members of the staff would not be able to tell the boys apart.

Following the separation surgery, the formerly quiet, laid-back Carl suddenly became awake and interactive. With a smile that rivaled his brother's, he began hogging the attention that had previously been showered on Clarence.

And Clarence's medical problems seemed to melt away. Following separation, it became possible to maintain his blood pressure in a normal range without the use of any medications at all. I proudly told Drs. Goodrich and Staffenberg that by separating Carl and Clarence, they had apparently accidentally stumbled on an effective cure for hypertension; the only problem was that in order for this cure to work, you had to be hypertensive and a conjoined twin! For some reason, neither doctor laughed.

But the resolution of his hypertension wasn't the only change that occurred in Clarence. In addition, his appetite improved and he began gaining weight. With the added weight, which caused his face to fill out, and the adoption of a frequent smile by Carl, it became difficult to tell the boys apart (a task that had been easy prior to the separation).

How to explain all this? In retrospect, Dr. Goodrich's theory appeared to be correct: Clarence had served as the pump twin for Carl, sending blood into his brother's cerebral circulation and then draining it back to his own heart. Following separation, Clarence only had to supply blood to his own circulatory system; the decrease in cardiac responsibility led to his blood pressure, which had been so high in order to perfuse Carl's circulation, to return to normal; also, he no longer needed to expend extra calories on the twofold work his heart was doing; with the decrease in his basal metabolic rate, he was able to gain weight without significantly increasing his caloric intake. And Carl, now no longer reliant on his brother for blood flow, was doing a better job of perfusing his own brain, leading to the awakening of his personality.

In the weeks following the surgery, Drs. Staffenberg and Goodrich became international celebrities. The surgeons were featured on network news programs and invited to speak at international meetings. Because of its apparent success, the Goodrich procedure has become the accepted standard method of separating craniopagus conjoined twins.

On October 13, 2004, Michael R. Bloomberg, the mayor of New York, presented a Special Recognition Award to CHAM and the entire team for the spectacular surgery Drs. Goodrich and Staffenberg had performed. And in its special "Best (and Worst) of 2004" issue, *People* magazine cited the separation of the Aguirre twins as one of the major events of the year.

BECAUSE CARL AND CLARENCE had spent so much time lying on their backs, they had little strength in the muscles of their trunks and limbs. Before they would be able to sit or walk, it would be necessary to strengthen those muscles. Their therapy regimen was beefed up. And slowly they made progress.

Within weeks of resuming therapy following recovery from the separation surgery, the twins were able to sit without assistance. Within two months, they were able to stand for short periods. By late February 2005, the day I walked onto the second floor of Blythedale, they were riding tricycles. And late that summer, around the first anniversary of their final surgery, Clarence independently took a few steps toward his mother, who was waiting for him outside Therapy Village at Garwood. It was the first time either boy had taken a step on his own.

Being involved in the care of Carl and Clarence has been the most gratifying experience in my medical career. From working with these remarkable boys and their even more remarkable mother—and alongside a team of brilliant and creative people—I've learned that virtually anything is possible in medicine, that no matter how difficult or unlikely a situation might be, with hard work, perseverance, and persistence, miracles can happen.

Postscript

SINCE THIS ESSAY was written, many events have occurred in the lives of Carl and Clarence Aguirre. In the early spring of 2007, just before the twins celebrated their fifth birthdays, Arlene and her sons left Garwood, which had been their home since their arrival from the Philippines in 2004. Through the work of the family's amazing social worker, Meredith Gosin, and some of their friends, the Aguirres were able to move into a two-bedroom house in Scarsdale, New York. Here, Arlene and her sons could, for the first time, live as a family rather than as patients in a long-term care facility.

In the fall of 2007, the boys began kindergarten. Although Clarence has developed nicely, Carl has had some issues; he has weakness on his right side that is being treated with therapy. Also, in the days following the separation, Carl had a seizure, a not unusual consequence of the trauma his brain underwent during the surgery. Carl's seizures increased in number in the months following separation, so one of our neurologists began him on an anticonvulsant medication. Although the anticonvulsants have stopped the seizures, Carl has suffered some adverse effects: he is clearly developmentally slower than his brother, lagging behind as his brother continues to make progress.

For a long time after the separation surgery, neither boy spoke. Their lack of speech was troubling to those of us who cared for them: as I've already noted, we could accept the fact that they were delayed in attainment of their motor skills; after all, while conjoined, there was no way they could sit up or stand or walk. But this should not have impaired their ability to reach cognitive milestones.

In trying to explain their lack of speech, I keep coming back to the fact that during the surgery, Dr. Goodrich discovered that their brains weren't completely separate. Is it possible that while joined together, the boys were communicating through impulses conducted through this conjoined portion of their brain, silently "talking" to each other without words? Could this be the answer to why, both prior to and in the months following the final surgery, they never said a word?

Unfortunately, because we didn't know about the shared portion of their brains until too late, until after it would have been possible to do studies to examine this possibility, we have no way of knowing the answers to these questions. (Of course, had we known beforehand that the boys shared a portion of their cerebral cortex, there's a good chance that Dr. Goodrich never would have taken on the challenge of separating the Aguirres in the first place!)

The boys still have a long way to go. As can be seen in the photo below from their sixth birthday party, they are still wearing helmets to protect their brains from injury. At the time of the separation, there wasn't enough bone to provide complete skulls for both Carl and Clarence. Imaging studies have

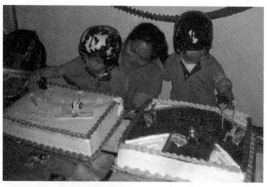

The twins at their sixth birthday party, April 20, 2008. Carl is at the left, Arlene is in the middle, and Clarence is at the right. (Photo by Jim Goodrich)

demonstrated that both boys have generated additional bone, but ultimately, using either bone harvested from other parts of their bodies (such as from their hips or ribs) or artificial bone (made from bars of a substance called hydroxyapatite), they will need to undergo surgery to reconstruct their skulls.

I've talked a lot with Arlene about the future. Although she has faced many problems since the separation of her sons, she has never regretted anything that's happened, any decision she's made.

"Dr. Goodrich saved my sons' lives," she says. "From the beginning, I told him that all I wanted was to have two separate boys. He did that for me, he gave me that. My boys are a miracle. They are two miracles."

CHAPTER 16

Three Pictures

"DEAR DR. MARION," the e-mail message began, "I'm sorry about the quality of these pictures. I took them with my cell phone. But I think that when you see them, you'll understand why I'm sending them."

The e-mail, with its three attachments, had come from Marcia G., the mother of Alena, a seven-year-old girl I'd been following for the past five years. As I clicked the button that would open the first attachment and waited for it to load on my very slow computer, I thought back to the first time I'd met Alena and her parents.

IT WAS MID-DECEMBER 2002. Although the family had been referred by Alena's pediatrician, the recommendation for the appointment had actually come from the child's cardiologist. Over the course of the previous six weeks, Alena had been evaluated by this cardiologist, as well as by an endocrinologist and an otolaryngologist (an ear, nose throat specialist, or

ENT) for problems relating to each one's specialty: the ENT had seen her because of delayed speech, chronic ear infections, and mild hearing loss; the cardiologist had been asked by the pediatrician to evaluate her heart murmur; and the endocrinologist had been called in to come up with an explanation and treatment for her extremely short stature. Each physician had made attempts to diagnose and treat these specific problems. However, in addition, after performing an echocardiogram that showed that it was stenosis of the mitral and aortic valves that was causing the girl's heart murmur, the cardiologist had reported back to the pediatrician that he felt that there was something else going on with this child, some other condition on which he could not put his finger, something that was causing the problem he'd been asked to evaluate. He had suggested that perhaps a medical geneticist should see her. And so, Marcia had been given my name and told to call me to set up an appointment.

The cardiologist had been right: there clearly was something wrong with Alena. While walking down the hall from the waiting area to my exam room with Alena and her mother, seeing the girl's mildly coarsened facial features; her thickened, clawlike hands; and her slightly stooped posture, I was able to tell what that something else was. Even before making it to the room, I knew that Alena, like Thomas Sweeney and Erin Wood, almost certainly had a mucopolysaccharidosis. And as had been the case with Thomas, by knowing this information, I felt I could pretty much predict what this little girl's future was going to be like. So as we walked, I began to organize the words that I would have to say to this girl's parents, the horrible information I'd have to impart to them over the course of the next hour, facts that were sure to forever change the course of their lives.

After settling the family into the exam room, I began to take the history. Alena's story was unusual and compelling, making this tragedy even sadder. Born in Siberia, she'd lived with her biological parents until the age of 17 months, when, for reasons that will never be known to us, she was abandoned by them and placed in an orphanage. Alena became one of about 50 parentless children living in cribs on an open ward in that large, cold institution. Chances were that, once admitted to this place, the girl would spend the better part of her childhood there, getting out only when she finally reached the age at which she'd be able to care for herself.

But then, the first of a series of miracles that would touch Alena's life occurred. A few months after she'd arrived at the orphanage, thousands of miles away, Marcia and her husband, Alex, began viewing videotapes of children available for adoption from orphanages around the world. Marcia and Alex were childless; although they had tried for years to have a baby of their own, Marcia had never become pregnant. Multiple evaluations had failed to identify a cause for their infertility; multiple new and innovative treatments had failed to solve it. Ultimately, the couple had given up, coming to terms with the fact that they would never become pregnant, eventually coming to the conclusion that adoption was their only option.

It was while viewing those videotapes, produced by institutions in Russia, China, Ecuador, and other countries, that Marcia saw Alena; it was love at first sight. The woman couldn't take her eyes off this little girl. Having seen that video myself, I can understand why Marcia reacted like this: dolled up in a gold party dress, with her long blond hair flowing behind her, Alena was definitely the belle of the orphanage. Vivacious and outgoing, she appeared in scene after scene interacting with other children, playing with toys, or just running around in circles. In every case, she was always the center of attention, the child on whom one's eyes naturally fixed. It was her smile that caused this reaction, so bright it lit up the room. After seeing the tape only once, Marcia was hooked: she vowed that as soon as she was able to arrange it, she'd go to Siberia, travel to that orphanage, meet that little girl, and bring her girl home.

Having watched that videotape a few times now, I've been struck by two additional facts about Alena. First, there's a definite resemblance between Alena and Marcia, a similarity in hair and skin coloring, in their size (both are petite), and in their body shape. Undoubtedly, this resemblance was one of the facts that drew this adoptive mother to this adoptive child in the first place: the girl looked as if she could have been the woman's biological daughter.

Also apparent from viewing that videotape is the fact that even at 17 months of age, Alena already showed some of the physical signs of a mucopolysaccharidosis. Though the signs are subtle, her face shows the slight coarsening, her hands the slight thickening that are characteristic of the early stages of these disorders. Since viewing the videotape, I've wondered if Alena's biological parents might have also recognized these characteristic signs, features of an autosomal recessively inherited genetic disorder that may well have been present in one or more of their previous children. Perhaps they recognized these early signs, realized that Alena was affected, and rather than subjecting themselves to the horrible future that was the inevitable consequence of her condition, they opted to turn over this beautiful toddler to the orphanage at which Marcia and Alex ultimately found her.

As soon as they viewed the video, Marcia and Alex began the process of adopting Alena. They filled out paperwork, consulted with attorneys and pediatricians who are experts in international adoption, paid everyone involved a hefty fee. Finally, when all was arranged, they traveled to Siberia, where at last they met the little girl in person.

They were not disappointed. Within four weeks, the couple was back in Westchester County with their new daughter. Alena, just shy of her second birthday when the jet landed at Kennedy airport, instantaneously adjusted to her new life of luxury. Talk about culture shock! After spending months on the ward of the orphanage with little personal contact, no privacy, and virtually no possessions to call her own, she was now living in a home where she had her own room, her own bed, all the toys and games she could imagine or wish for, and the constant attention of a pair of loving and doting parents. Although she spoke no English, limiting her ability to communicate with anyone, and, for the second time, had left the place that had been her home, she warmed immediately to her adoptive parents and settled right in.

Soon after her arrival, Marcia and Alex took Alena to a pediatrician, who, upon examining her, had noted the heart murmur and referred her to the cardiologist who ultimately requested that the girl be referred to a geneticist. That had led them to my office, and what I knew was going to be a horrible visit.

I took this history from Marcia and Alex and then examined the girl; nothing I found on that examination dissuaded me from the diagnosis on which I had fixed on the short walk from the waiting room. And so, after Marcia had dressed her daughter and placed her on her lap on one of the chairs in the exam room, I closed my eyes and launched into what is always the most painful discussion any physician can have with the parents of a child.

"As you know," I began telling Marcia and Alex, "Alena was sent to me because of the problems her other doctors identified. What clinical geneticists do is treat the problems like pieces of a puzzle and try to assemble them into a single diagnosis. Alena has fluid in her middle ears that has led to some hearing loss and speech delay; she has a heart murmur that the cardiologist found to be due to some thickening of her heart valves; she's very short, but her level of growth hormone has been found to be normal. The question is, Do these problems exist in isolation, or are they all part of a single condition?"

Marcia interrupted me. "But, Dr. Marion, Alena has spent the last six months living under terrible conditions. She hasn't had enough good food; wouldn't that have caused her to grow poorly? And she's lived with 50 other kids on a ward in Siberia that never had enough heat; wouldn't that cause her to have ear infections and get fluid in her ears? And of course her speech is delayed: until six weeks ago, she was living in a place where no one spoke English, and she has come to a place where no one speaks Russian. Isn't the change in language reason enough for her to be delayed?"

I agreed with the mother that all of these were possible explanations, but then, firmly, I went on. "My examination also shows some subtle findings that we can't explain on the basis of her having lived in an orphanage. For instance, her facial features are a little thickened—"

"Thickened?" Marcia asked. "What does that mean? I've never heard of someone's face being thick."

"And her hands are also thickened," I continued. "Also, her joints are stiffer than I would expect for a child of her age."

"Stiff joints?" Alex asked. "You mean like in arthritis?"

I nodded and went on. "From all of this, I think Alena may have one of a group of conditions known as the mucopolysaccharidoses, or MPSs for short. In the MPSs, the cells that form the body are missing an enzyme that's needed to break down complex chemicals. If this enzyme is missing, the chemicals build up in the bloodstream and get deposited in the connective tissue, the heart, the bones, the joints, and in many cases the brain—"

"You can tell this by looking at her for ten minutes?" Alex asked.

"I'm not sure she has it," I responded. "We need to do some tests. But this would explain a lot of the things that have been happening to Alena."

Marcia replied, "Not to contradict you—I know our other doctors think very highly of you—but I think you're wrong about this. I think that Alena has all these problems because of the conditions under which she's been living. But for argument's sake, let's say she does have one these MPSs. What's the treatment?"

"Let's not get ahead of ourselves," I said. "Before we start talking about possible therapies, let's see if she really has it."

"No, before we go any further, I need to know: what's the treatment for this muco-whatever?"

I hesitated. "There's currently no treatment for any of the mucopolysaccharidoses," I continued. "If she does have one of these disorders, her organs will slowly accumulate more and more of these chemicals."

"No treatment?" Marcia said as tears began forming in her eyes. "You mean she's going to die of this?"

I didn't say anything. I bit my lip and looked on as both parents dissolved into tears.

"I'm not 100 percent sure of the diagnosis," I said again after a while had passed, fighting off my own tears. "Before we start worrying about what's going to happen, let's see what the tests show."

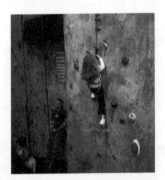 THE FIRST ATTACHMENT finally opened, and a photo appeared on my computer screen. I immediately agreed with Marcia's assessments, both about the picture's quality and about its significance. The grainy photo showed the back of a little girl with long blond hair, dangling from a rope near the bottom of a climbing wall. The dangling girl was Alena; from conversations with her and her

mother, I knew she'd been trying to climb to the top of this wall, located in a park near her family's home, for nearly six months now. But due to the worsening tightness of her joints and her decreased stamina, both consequences of her underlying condition, she had thus far failed in this quest. Could these photos be evidence that the kid had finally reached this goal?

Hopefully, I clicked the button for the second attachment and again waited for a photo to load.

AFTER DELIVERING THE terrible news that I suspected that Alena had an incurable, progressive disease to Alex and Marcia that day in December 2002, I sent the girl off to get some diagnostic tests done. The X-rays performed at Children's Hospital showed that Alena's bones were packed with stored material; I could tell from looking at a single lateral view of her spine that my hunch was correct, and the radiologist confirmed this, reporting that there were "classic signs of dysostosis multiplex, consistent with the diagnosis of a mucopolysaccharidosis." The urine we sent also was abnormal, showing a marked excess in the amount of a chemical called dermatan sulfate; a sample of blood sent to the New York State lab on Staten Island revealed that Alena's cells were lacking the enzyme arylsulfatase B (also called N-acetylgalactosamine-4-sulfatase), confirming that Alena had mucopolysaccharidosis type VI, or as it's more commonly called, Maroteaux-Lamy syndrome.

So, two weeks after the initial visit, I was again sitting with Marcia in an exam room on the fifth floor of Children's Hospital. Following my instructions, she had left Alena at home with a baby-sitter. (Alex had had to go to work that day, so Marcia had come by herself.) As soon as she sat down, I told her the results of the testing.

"How could this have happened?" Marcia pleaded with me. She was extremely angry and clearly very sad. "I had the medical records reviewed by some of the top specialists in the field of international adoption in the United States. We had doctors' reports, people reviewed those videotapes, no one told us there was even a chance of a problem! How can this be?"

"Alena's features are subtle," I replied. "Unless you have special training in genetics, you probably wouldn't pick them up. The thing to remember, the good news in this case, is that unlike most of the other MPSs, Maroteaux-Lamy syndrome doesn't cause involvement of the brain. She'll have normal intelligence; she'll be able to go to school, have friends, do things other kids do, and—"

"What good will normal intelligence be to her if she's going to die before she reaches 18?" Marcia interrupted, with tears in her eyes. "To tell you the truth, knowing what's going to happen to her, I believe she'd be better off if she became retarded and didn't know what was going on."

We were quiet for a minute. I had no response to her comment. Then, as if pleading with me, Marcia said, "And there's no treatment for this condition? How is it possible that there's no treatment? This is America! There are treatments for everything."

"There is some research going on to find a way to replace the enzyme that's missing in the bloodstream of people with Maroteaux-Lamy syndrome," I replied. "There's nothing available yet, but in a few years—"

"A few years will be too late!" Marcia interrupted again, pleading. "From what I read on the Internet, every day this girl's body is getting more and more choked by these chemicals. I don't have time to wait." She broke into tears.

Wiping the tears from my own eyes, I put my hand on her shoulder, trying to comfort her.

"I can't do this," Marcia finally said to me. "I can't live like this. Dr. Marion, when I was seven, my older brother got leukemia. The doctors who took care of him told my parents the same thing you're telling us, that there was no treatment but that in a few years there might be something that would come along to help him. It took my brother two years to die, and in that time absolutely nothing became available. It was terrible watching him suffer every day, knowing there was nothing anyone could do to help him. His illness and death destroyed my parents and their marriage. I can't go through this. I can't sit by and watch my child suffer and die like my brother did. I just can't do it." She began crying again.

I was quiet. Finally, I said, "Ms. G., there's only a limited number of choices here—"

"Dr. Marion," she cut in, "I brought Alena to this country and into my home to give her a better life. I didn't bring her here so that I could watch her get sicker and sicker until she finally dies. I can't live with this. I can't live like this. How about if I put her in foster care? She could go with a family who would take care of her and love her. I would be involved in helping them take care of her, like I was her aunt or her cousin, something like that. I just can't deal with this every day of my life, having her in my house, watching her get sicker and sicker day after day after day."

My sympathy for this woman turned to hostility. How could she even think of saying these things about her daughter? Alena was a little girl, a child who, because of her condition, was going to need a lot of help and a lot of love as she traversed the very rocky course of the coming years; she was not some piece of merchandise, a sweater that could be returned to the department store because it was the wrong size or the wrong color, a coffee table that had to go back to the furniture store because it didn't fit in with the rest of the decor! As in marriages, adoptions are promises made for better or for worse, in sickness and in health, until death breaks the bond. Unlike marriages, however, these promises between parent and child should not be negotiable or breakable, even if the adoptee happens to have a serious illness.

I was angry, but I managed to keep my anger in check because, having now met this woman on two occasions, I knew three additional facts about her and about the condition that affected Alena. First, I knew that Marcia, like most people who hear bad news, was functioning on pure emotions: she was hurting, she was angry and very sad, and she was not putting any thought into the consequences of her words. Second, from watching her interact with Alena during the first visit, I knew that she and her husband loved this little girl very much; giving her up after she'd lived as their daughter in their home now for more than two months would be nearly impossible. Third, having been keeping up on research developments, I knew that a Phase 1 clinical trial of enzyme replacement therapy for Maroteaux-Lamy syndrome had recently ended with good results, and that a Phase 2 trial was already under way.

Undoubtedly, a treatment for this condition was only a couple of years down the road.

FINALLY, THE SECOND attachment sent to me by Marcia opened on my computer, and another, equally grainy photo appeared on the screen.

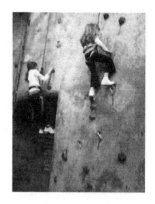

This picture also showed Alena from the rear, this time about 12 feet above the ground. Her feet are planted in the wall's toeholds; her left hand and arm are wrapped tightly around a rope; her right hand is digging into the wall for support. She is concentrating all of her effort on the climb.

I'd seen pictures of Alena like this before. In the past, though, this had been about the maximum height she'd been able to reach. I found myself anticipating what the third attachment might show. I clicked the button and once again waited for the photo to load.

THE DEVELOPMENT OF a new drug is expensive, incredibly hard, and enormously time-consuming. When the drug is a treatment for a condition that is common (meaning that the drug will be sought after and therefore likely to make a large profit), pharmaceutical companies are more than willing to spend the money, put up with the aggravation imposed by oversight agencies, and ultimately bear the burden of bringing the drug to market. But what about drugs that are being developed for conditions that are so rare that it's difficult to find enough affected individuals to even test the drug's efficacy, drugs that are likely to never be profitable?

MPS VI, the condition originally described in 1963 by Pierre Maroteaux and Maurice Lamy, two French pediatricians, is a rare condition. Because it occurs in only 2 or 3 individuals per 1 million, most pediatricians go through their entire careers without seeing a single affected patient. Any drug developed for such a rare disorder would never, ever reach a point at which it would be profitable for the pharmaceutical company. So why even pursue a treatment?

The answer lies in one of the important characteristics of this condition: unlike most of the other MPSs, such as Hunter and Sanfilippo syndromes, Maroteaux-Lamy affects the viscera, the heart and lungs, the joints and bones, the facial structures and the airway, but spares the central nervous system: levels of arylsulfatase B in the brain and cerebrospinal fluid are normal. Therefore, development of an effective treatment would not have to solve the problem of getting a large protein across the blood-brain barrier. So, although MPS VI is rare, developing an enzyme replacement therapy might lead the way to treatments for other, much more common (and therefore more profitable) conditions.

With this in mind, BioMarin, a pharmaceutical company based in California, developed Naglazyme (galsulfase), a product that contains a form of arylsulfatase B. Before being approved by the Food and Drug Administration for use in humans, drugs in development must go through three phases of clinical trials: Phase 1, in which the drug is tested in a small group of patients (20–80) to check that it's safe, to determine a reasonable dosage range, and to identify any side effects; Phase 2, in which the drug is used in a larger group of patients to see if it's effective and to further evaluate its safety; and Phase 3, in which the drug is given to large groups of patients to further determine its effectiveness, monitor side effects, compare it to other treatments that are available, and collect information that will allow the drug to be used safely. At the time of Alena's diagnosis, the efficacy of Naglazyme had already been demonstrated in a Phase 1 trial, and Phase 2 trials were under way and nearing completion. Since each phase lasts for approximately one to one and a half years, I estimated that treatment to arrest the progression of Alena's disease was probably two to three years away. It was just a matter of the family hanging on.

SO, RATHER THAN showing my anger at Marcia and lecturing her about the fact that it was her responsibility to love and care for Alena no matter what, I laid back, responding to her questions and setting out the options. I told her that, as I saw it, there were basically two things she and her husband could choose to do: one was to put Alena into foster care and eventually allow her to be adopted by another family in the United States; the second option was for them to continue to care for her, love her, and treat her as their daughter. I made sure to tell her that any decision they made that was right for them was the correct one, that they should not be swayed by what anyone else—including other doctors, family members, or friends—might say; I told her that regardless of their decision, I'd be there to help them and support them in any way I could;

and, most important, I told her to avoid making a rash decision based on emotions and to instead take her time and carefully consider all the options.

I urged her to take her time in making this decision because I knew what was going to happen: with each passing day, Marcia and Alex would come to love Alena more; the more they loved her, the less likely it would be that they'd place her in foster care. My strategy worked: in early February, less than a month after the meeting at which I told Marcia of Alena's diagnosis—after Marcia had contacted the adoption agency she'd used and the international adoption experts she'd consulted, threatening to sue everyone involved, and after she'd contacted a foster care agency to find out the protocol for placing a child—she called my office: "We've decided to keep Alena," she told me. "Although we're still incredibly angry, we love this kid too much to give her up."

"You're making the right decision," I told her, even though as a geneticist I am never supposed to tell parents that their decisions are either right or wrong.

FOR THE NEXT few years I followed Alena closely, seeing her in my office every other month, watching helplessly as the storage of mucopolysaccharides in her body slowly but steadily robbed her of the ability to function. Because of the effect of the chemicals packed into her bones, the girl grew extremely slowly, falling further and further off the growth curve. Her joints became stiffer, her hands becoming so clawlike that she began having trouble gripping small toys. And her stamina diminished; I could see how limited she was becoming by just walking behind her on the short trek from the waiting area to the exam room. And although her parents, now fully devoted to their daughter and her special problems, coped with the deterioration as best they could, and together, in an attempt to keep her joints as limber as possible, we worked to get her as many sessions of physical and occupational therapy as possible, we each watched the Internet for information about the progression of the clinical trials for Naglazyme. The Phase 2 trial ended with success equal to that seen in Phase 1.[1] In 2004, when it was announced that the Phase 3 trial would soon be getting under way, Marcia called Dr. Paul Harmatz, a gastroenterologist at Oakland Children's Hospital who was one of the principal investigators in the study, and asked if Alena could be enrolled. Although she didn't like the idea of her daughter being a guinea pig, she realized that the sooner Alena was started on the enzyme replacement therapy, the better off she would be. Unfortunately, Dr. Harmatz's response was not positive: the rules of the clinical trial stated that those involved had to be age seven or older, and Alena was not even close. Although we both argued and begged, the rules were sacrosanct; Alena would have to wait for the drug's final approval.

That approval finally came from the Food and Drug Administration on May 31, 2005, following the report of the efficacy and safety of Naglazyme by the Phase 3 study group, and BioMarin received approval to market the drug on June 1. By the end of June, all arrangements had been made for Alena to receive Naglazyme for the first time.

And then it happened. On a morning in early July 2005, Alex and Marcia brought Alena to Children's Hospital for that first treatment. Naglazyme is tricky; it has to be given slowly, over a three- to four-hour period, by intravenous infusion; during the infusion, in order to monitor for any serious side effects, vital signs need to be monitored every 15 minutes.

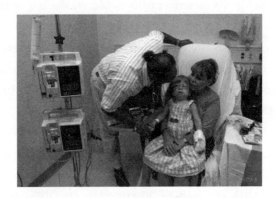

This photo, taken just before my colleague, Dr. Paul Levy, began her IV, shows how frightened Alena looked before that first treatment. But once the needle was in and the medication was flowing, she relaxed, realizing that it didn't hurt at all. The photo below shows her later during that infusion.

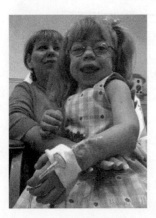

Alena was the first patient in the northeastern United States (other than those enrolled in the trials) treated with Naglazyme. Since that first infusion, her parents have brought her back to the hospital every Tuesday morning for repeat treatments; during the entire year she's been receiving infusions, there has been not a single adverse reaction. And Dr. Levy and I have stood back and watched, amazed, at the progress she's made: in the first three months of treatment, Alena grew a whopping four inches; her joints were perceptively more mobile, and she didn't get tired or winded walking from the waiting room to the exam room. Her progress has been almost miraculous.

Just as these thoughts were going through my mind, the third image appeared on my screen. And there she was!

I began smiling as soon as I saw it; pretty soon, tears were form-ing in my eyes. The photo showed Alena at the top of the wall. But rather than facing the wall, the lit-tle girl, still holding on with all her might, had now turned her body slightly to face her mother. She was looking back over her right shoulder; on her face, she flashed 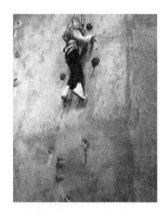 a huge smile. After all that time, after all those attempts, after all that hard work she'd put in with her therapists and all the poking and prodding she'd put up with every Tuesday morning for the past year, she'd finally made it!

What had happened in this park in northern Westchester County was truly a miracle. For Alena to reach the top of that climbing wall, a staggering cascade of events had to happen in precisely the right order. Had she been born just ten years earlier, there would have been no Naglazyme available to stop the progression of her disease. Had her biological parents not abandoned her, had she lived her entire life with them in

Siberia, she'd never have had the opportunity to receive the proper medication. Had she not been in that orphanage at the time those videotapes were being made, Alex and Marcia would never have seen her face, never fallen in love with her, and never brought her back to New York. Had the couple not been looking to adopt a daughter at just that time, Alena would have been passed over. Alena's life has been a cosmic event, the lining up of seemingly impossible factors in just the right order to allow her to be one of the first ones on earth to benefit from a major scientific breakthrough.

I'm often asked why in God's name I chose to become a geneticist. After all, what with trisomy 13 and other chromosome abnormalities, the mucopolysaccharidoses and other metabolic diseases, and so many other conditions, the prognosis of my patients is so poor, and the treatments often non-existent; day after day the news is bad. But the answer is clear: it is because of Alena that I became a geneticist; because of Alena and Carl and Clarence and so many other kids like these three whose lives are made better, even a little bit better, by my involvement. For me, this is much more than I deserve. I have definitely chosen the right career; and for sure, I'm fortunate to be able to perform this work with the patients whose lives are chronicled in these essays, as well as so many others whose stories do not appear here.

AFTERWORD

I STARTED MEDICAL SCHOOL in the Bronx in August 1975. Although I escaped to Boston from July 1979 until June 1980 to do my internship at the Boston Floating Hospital, I returned to the Bronx for my residency and fellowship, and joined the faculty at the Albert Einstein College of Medicine at the completion of my training. As I write this, except for that one year in Boston, I've spent 34 years working in this borough.

One advantage of staying on at the same institution for so many years is that you never get the sense that you're getting older; I find that I'm still surrounded by the people who educated me, people who themselves don't look any older than they did when I first met them (although this is obviously just an illusion). The net effect of this is that I have the sense that I haven't aged at all either; walking around campus, interacting with medical students, I feel like I'm still a medical student myself. This is fine most of the time, but occasionally reality breaks through. This happened a few years ago in one of the medical school's classrooms.

It was early winter and the first-year students were struggling through the second month of the required Molecular and

Cellular Foundations in Medicine course. I was sitting at the front of the room, precepting a Clinical Case Conference, a session designed to integrate principles of basic and clinical sciences. Surrounding me were 20 eager students who had assembled their desks in a rectangle. After introducing myself and announcing that the topic for that day's discussion was diabetes mellitus, I asked for a volunteer to begin presenting the case described on the handout they'd all received the day before. After raising his hand, Lev, one of the most eager of the students, began to speak.

The case involved a 58-year-old man who, after a bout of pneumonia, developed polyuria, polydipsia, and polyphagia (i.e., he was peeing too much, drinking too much, and eating too much). While Lev began to describe the man's initial history, I scanned the room, looking at the students' faces. My attention was snagged by the young man sitting immediately to my left; a tall, sturdy-appearing fellow, he'd entered the room late and, unlike the other students, had neglected to put his name card (designed so that the preceptor could call on students when their eagerness began to lag) on the desk in front of him. There was something familiar about this young man, something that made me think that I'd seen him someplace before. As Lev continued, I tried my best to come up with where. Had I interviewed him when he'd been applying to medical school the year before? I didn't think so. Had he spoken with me after one of my lectures to the first-year class? No, I'm sure his image wouldn't have sunk into my consciousness so indelibly with such brief contact.

Interrupting my reverie, I tried to focus on the case at hand.

"Does anyone have any idea what the significance of this man's excessive drinking is?" I asked. "And why has he lost eight pounds if he's been eating as much as he says he has?" When a few seconds had passed and no volunteer had emerged from the group, I began to scan the roster of names I'd been given for a victim. As soon as I saw the name "Jonathan Klein," the bell in my head began to ring.

IT WAS THE late fall of 1978, and Beth and I were standing in the living room of an apartment in one of the housing towers in which medical students lived. As co-editor of our class's yearbook, it was my responsibility to take photographs of all my classmates. During our rounds that evening, we were taking the senior picture of Michael Klein and his family.

Michael was one of the few members of our class who had a child; his son, Jonathan, was then about a year old. For the photo shoot Jonathan, who was very well behaved for a kid of his age, had been neatly dressed in a navy blue sailor suit. While Beth shot the picture, Jonathan sat contentedly on his mother's lap, while his father, seated next to his wife, cradled the boy's legs.

Was it possible that that little boy in the sailor suit had become this strapping young man sitting in a Clinical Case Conference? Could it be that the son of one of my classmates was old enough to be a first-year student at the medical school his father and I had attended? No, it didn't seem possible; after all, I still felt like a medical student myself. But as I sat in that room, I started to do the math and realized that it was not only possible but actually probable.

HAVING BEEN BLOWN away by this epiphany, having completely lost my train of thought, I found it difficult to go on without interrupting the small group session. Luckily for me, Jennifer, one of the other students in the room, had begun to answer the questions I'd posed before I'd drifted back to 1978, and, although I hadn't been paying attention, it seemed as if she had offered a cogent and well-thought-out response. When she finished, before another student could begin to speak, I asked (already knowing the answer), "Where is Jonathan Klein?"

As I expected, the young man immediately to my left raised his hand.

"Are you Michael Klein's son?" I asked.

"Yeah," he responded. "How do you know my dad?"

"We were medical school classmates," I answered. "I remember you as a little boy. My wife and I took your picture for our class's yearbook."

"The one of me in the sailor suit?" he asked, and I nodded. "I hated that sailor suit," he continued. "My mother used to make me wear it for all formal occasions. It made me look like a real geek."

"No, you were cute," I said. "You were very cute. And now you're an Einstein student."

He nodded.

There followed an uncomfortable silence. Having completely derailed the educational exercise with my own agenda, I realized that I had to do something fast to get us back on track. "You guys don't understand the significance of this," I began, addressing the whole group, unsure of exactly where I was heading. "Meeting me for the first time, you all probably think of me as an old fart." (There was snickering.) "And I probably am an old fart." (The snickering intensified.) "But because I've spent my entire career at this medical school, I have this weird sense that I've never gotten older, that I'm actually your contemporary. By having Jonathan in this class, I have to accept the fact that I'm not a first-year medical student anymore, that I'm actually old enough to have a child who's a first-year medical student. That's pretty sobering!"

In the next few moments, there again was an uncomfortable silence in the room. Finally, Lev spoke up: "Dr. Marion, now that you're done having your midlife crisis, should I go on reading the case?"

I smiled and nodded, and he continued presenting the case of the 58-year-old man with diabetes.

The presence of Jonathan in that class forever shattered my own warped impression that I was still a contemporary of first-year medical students. But although I've gotten over that illusion, I still have a great deal of trouble coming to grips with the fact that I'm now considered a "senior faculty member." I still feel uncomfortable when students and residents (and even recently, young faculty members) call me "Dr. Marion." I'm always turning around, expecting my older brother (who's the "real" Dr. Marion) to be standing there. I guess this is one of the things about growing older in the Bronx with which I'll never feel comfortable.

THE 35 YEARS I'VE spent at Einstein represent more than half of the entire history of the field of modern genetics, which officially began on April 25, 1953, when a one-page article by James

Watson and Francis Crick entitled "Molecular Structure of Nucleic Acids: A Structure for Deoxyribose Nucleic Acid" appeared in *Nature*. In 1982, when I began my fellowship and became a clinical geneticist, the field was nothing more than a sleepy backwater of pediatrics: we could do amniocenteses and sonograms, looking at fetuses and trying to identify those with problems, but there was little we could do to help those with abnormalities; we could examine children and identify patterns of malformations, make diagnoses, order chromosome testing to look for large chromosome abnormalities like trisomy 21 (the cause of Down syndrome), but again, once those abnormalities were diagnosed, there was virtually nothing we could do to cure them.

But as the years have passed, clinical genetics has changed more than any other field in medicine. My sleepy backwater has become the site of a revolution, a series of dramatic changes spurred on by the success of the Human Genome Project, as well as by the birth and development of the field of translational research. And just look at what's happened during the time these essays were written: the genetic bases of disorders such as Pfeiffer syndrome, hypohidrotic ectodermal dysplasia, and spinal muscular atrophy have been discovered, opening the door to possible treatment options in the future; through bone marrow transplantation and enzyme replacement therapy, previously lethal diseases such as congenital erythropoeitic porphyria and Maroteaux-Lamy syndrome can be treated, if not cured; and through the ingenuity and genius of creative surgeons, two boys seemingly permanently joined together because of a simple error in embryogenesis can now lead separate, active, and productive lives.

And remember, all of this has happened within a 20-year period. What will the next 20 years bring? For sure, technology will allow us to screen the 20,000 genes present in every individual at the time of birth, allowing us to know all changes in the genetic code that might predispose people to diseases. This advance will forever change the way medicine is practiced, taking it from a field in which we wait for people to develop symptoms and signs before we can treat them to one in which the predisposition to disease will be known from the start and prevention will be accomplished through manipulating the environment before symptoms ever appear. Although still in its childhood, genetic therapy, altering the way genes are expressed, will become commonplace.

FOR MANY REASONS, clinical genetics is a unique specialty. Because the conditions we geneticists treat are so sensitive, the work we do is different in many ways from the work done by other physicians. It's my hope to provide through these essays an understanding of some of these differences: of how we support our patients both emotionally as well as physically, of how we provide care not only to the person with the disease but also to the parents, the siblings, the grandparents. and the extended family. We talk to these other patients, offer them counseling about risks to future progeny and hope for the future, reassure them that nothing that they did caused or would have prevented the problem from occurring in the first place; we attend funerals, weddings, and graduations. We reach out much further than other physicians do.

Even the way we approach our patients is different from

how other specialists do it. We solve mysteries using a combination of detective work, pockets of unusual knowledge, intuition and hunches (which aren't always correct), and a great deal of luck. To paraphrase Sherlock Holmes, we clinical geneticists have trained ourselves to see things, to view and interpret what others might have overlooked. It is this observing that often provides us with the opportunity to make diagnoses like acute intermittent porphyria or hypohidrotic ectodermal dysplasia.

In my opinion, we clinical geneticists are underused by our colleagues as consultants. There are so many examples of children whose lives would have been improved had they been sent for a genetics consultation. Had the doctor in the emergency room who was seeing Melissa Moore called for a genetics consult, the terrible tragedy that befell the Moore family would have been avoided; had Nicole Ludlow been referred to a geneticist years before, there's a good chance that the girl's porphyria would have been diagnosed sooner.

This is how I view my specialty. As I've written many times in these essays, a revolution has occurred in my chosen field, a revolution brought about through new technology that has altered (or will soon alter) the way all of medicine is practiced. But having witnessed these advances firsthand, this revolution has seemed more like an evolution, much like the way I've somehow gone from being a medical student to a senior faculty member during the very brief 35 years I've spent working in the Bronx! Through the years, having had the opportunity to work with people like Carl and Clarence Aguirre; Alena G.; A.C. Sheridan and his mother, Erin Wood; the Kennedys; and the Cohens, I feel extremely fortunate to have chosen the field I chose. What a time it has been to be a geneticist! And what a time it will be in the future!

PHOTO CREDITS

The photographs on pages 220, 224, 231, and 239 are by Alice Attie and appear by permission of the Montefiore Medical Center and Arlene Aguirre.

The photograph on page 243 appears by permission of James T. Goodrich, MD, PhD, and Arlene Aguirre.

The photographs on pages 252, 257, and 263 appear by permission of Marcia Galan.

The photographs on page 262 appear by permission of The Journal News and Marcia Galan.

ENDNOTES

CHAPTER 1. FAILING A.C.

1. C. M. Barone, R. Marion, A. Shanske, R. Argamaso, and R. Shprint-zen, Craniofacial, Limb and Abdominal Abnormalities in a Distinct Syndrome: Relation to the Spectrum of Pfeiffer Syndrome, Type 3," *American Journal of Medical Genetics* 45 (1993): 745

N. H. Robin, J. A. Scott, J. E. Arnold, J. A. Goldstein, B. B. Shilling, R. W. Marion, and M. M. Cohen Jr., "Favorable Prognosis for Children with Pfeiffer Syndrome Types 2 and 3: Implications for Classification," *American Journal of Medical Genetics* 75 (1998): 240–44

J. T. Goodrich and C. Hall, eds., *Craniofacial Anomalies: Growth and Development from a Surgical Perspective* (New York: Thieme, 1995).

CHAPTER 2. A CASE OF ABUSE

1. *New England Journal of Medicine* 339 (October 1, 1998): 947–52.

CHAPTER 7. RELICS

1. S. Lefebvre, L. Burglen, S. Reboullet, O. Clermont, P. Burlet, L. Viollet, B. Benichou, C. Cruaud, P. Millasseau, M. Zeviani, D. Le Paslier, J. Frezal, D. Cohen, J. Weissenbach, A. Munnich, and J. Melki, "Identification and Characterization of a Spinal Muscular Atrophy-Determining Gene," *Cell* 80 (1995): 155–65.

CHAPTER 9. THE CHRISTMAS PRESENT

1. A. Donnenfeld, letter to the editor, *American Journal of Medical Genetics* 72 (1997): 123.

CHAPTER 11. NO SWEAT!

1. J. Kere et al., "X-linked Anhidrotic (Hypohidrotic) Ectodermal Dysplasia Is Caused by Mutation in a Novel Transmembrane Protein," *Nature Genetics* 13 (1996): 409–16.

CHAPTER 12. THE SKELETON IN MR. ANDERSON'S CLOSET

1. A. B. Marfan, "Un cas de deformation congenitale des quatre membres, plus prononcee aux extremites, caracterisee par l'allongement des os avec un certain degre d'amincissement." *Bulletins et Mémoires de la Société Medicale des Hôpitaux de Paris* 13 (1896): 220–26.

2. J. Habashi, D. P. Judge, T. M. Holm, R. D. Cohn, B. L. Loeys, et al., "Losartan, an AT1 Antagonist, Prevents Aortic Aneurysm in a Mouse Model of Marfan Syndrome," *Science* 312, no. 5770 (April 2006): 117–12.

CHAPTER 13. THE RIGHT PLACE, THE RIGHT TIME

1. I. Macalpine and R. Hunter, "The 'Insanity' of King George III: A Classic Case of Porphyria" *British Medical Journal* 1 (1966): 65–71.

CHAPTER 16. THREE PICTURES

1. P. Harmatz, D. Ketteridge, et al., "Direct Comparison of Measures of Endurance, Mobility, and Joint Function During Enzyme-Replacement Therapy of Mucopolysaccharidosis VI [Maroteaux-Lamy syndrome]: Results After 48 Weeks in a Phase 2 Open-Label Clinical Study of Recombinant Human N-acetylgalactosamine 4-sulfatase," *Pediatrics* 115, no. 6 (June 2005): 681–89.